COOKING WITH CATS -

Favorite Recipes of Crazy Cat People and the Felines We Feast With

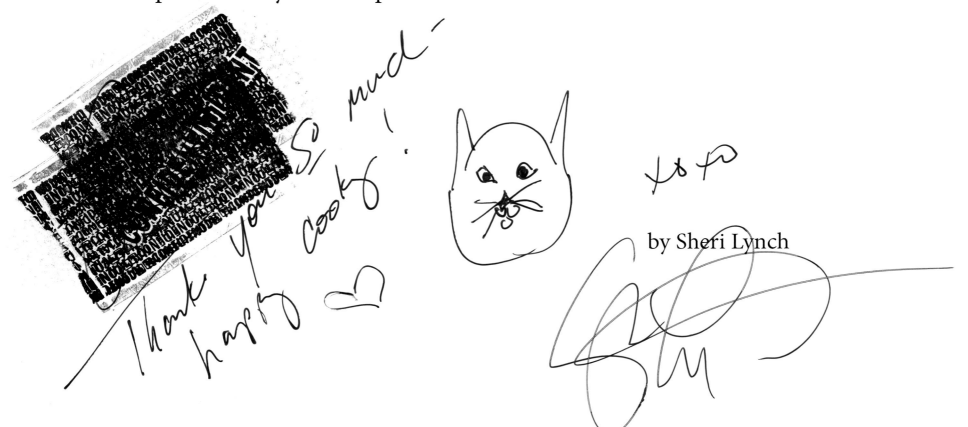

Thank you So much - happy cooky!

by Sheri Lynch

ISBN 978-1-950647-61-3

Publishing assistance by BookCrafters, Parker, Colorado.
www.bookcrafters.net

CATegories

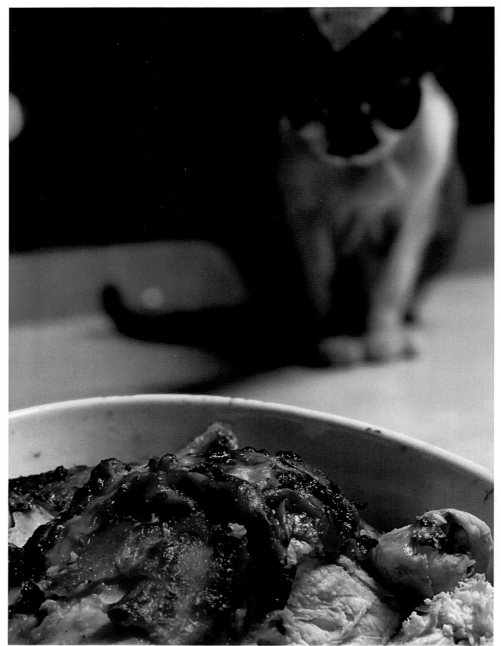
Photo Courtesy of Sheri Lynch

Introduction

The first thing I ever cooked all by myself was a batch of brownies in my Easy Bake Oven. "Batch" might be too strong a word for the small puck of underbaked chocolate goo I produced, but for an 8-year-old with only a 100-watt lightbulb to work with, it wasn't half bad. I loved that Easy Bake oven so very much. And I also loved cats, even though the first cat I remember our family having was a regal Siamese named Pywacket who worshipped my mother, loathed my father, and was mostly indifferent to me. I was determined to win her over. I came up with a brilliant plan: I'd prepare a special feast just for her. I mixed a tiny pan of dry and wet cat food and slid it into the Easy Bake Oven.

You wouldn't think a light bulb heating up some cat food could cause much of a problem, but that's where you're mistaken. We had to fling open every door and window and evacuate the house. In the dead of winter. In northern Wyoming. I learned quite a bit that day, including some colorful new language. From that point on, it was surely my destiny to one day whip up a novelty cookbook for crazy cat people.

Here's the thing: every cat lover I have ever known is also either a great cook or a very enthusiastic eater. Coincidence? I don't think so. To appreciate the beauty and mystery of the domestic cat, that fierce predator made somehow miniature and curled up at your side, purring, is to appreciate the sensual. And food is deeply sensual. This isn't a slam on dogs – I have several. It's just a different energy, a different way of moving through the world. Not everyone gets it. I've had people say to me, "Girl, with those cats walking around your kitchen, I'm not eating anything you're cooking." That's cool. I will say, in my own defense, I'm not cooking the cats themselves and I have a near-obsession with tidiness, but whatever. I'm not here to force feed anyone. But if you are a person who loves good food, make friends with a crazy cat lady or dude.

I come from a family of great cooks, and not one of them ever seemed to use a recipe. I learned how to cook by watching and by tasting and by feel. This strategy, however, does not work for baking, which is more chemistry than improv. It was baking that started my lifelong obsession with reading cookbooks. That's where I learned the why of what I'd watched my grandmothers and aunts doing in the kitchen. Why baking powder in one recipe, baking soda in another. How when spices are added is just as important as how much spice, or which. Cookbooks taught me the words for techniques I'd grown up taking for granted: braising, blooming, browning, caramelizing. The more I learned about "real" recipes, the more awed I was at how casually my grandmother could throw a beautiful scratch cake together while keeping one eye glued to her daytime soaps.

I love fancy meals and recipes created by gifted chefs, but my true heart belongs to the home cook. For this book, I reached out to lots of fellow cooking cat fanciers that I know and asked them to share a favorite recipe. There's even a little special nibble at the very end just for your cats. For novice cooks, I have two pieces of advice: don't be afraid to experiment. Food doesn't have to be perfect to be delicious. Second, get a kitchen scale and an instant-read thermometer. The first helps you measure precise quantities, often critical in baking, and the second takes the guesswork out of preparing meats. I have tons of gadgets and tools because Christmas comes every year and my family knows I love to cook. But you know what? I still mix things by hand, drag out the same pan or baking sheets that I've had forever, and use a juicer that I bought for $5 at a thrift store. Fancy tools are so fun to play with, but you can also make a feast with little more than your own two hands. Just trust me on the thermometer. It's a real game changer.

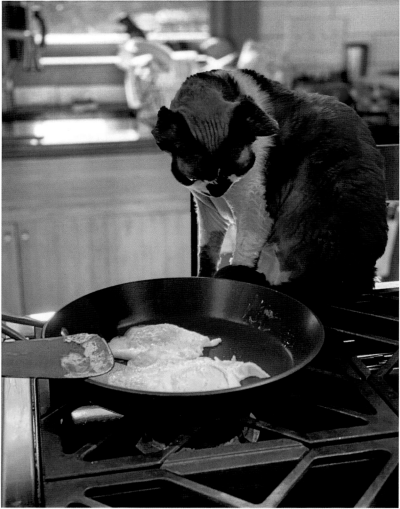

Photo Courtesy of Sheri Lynch

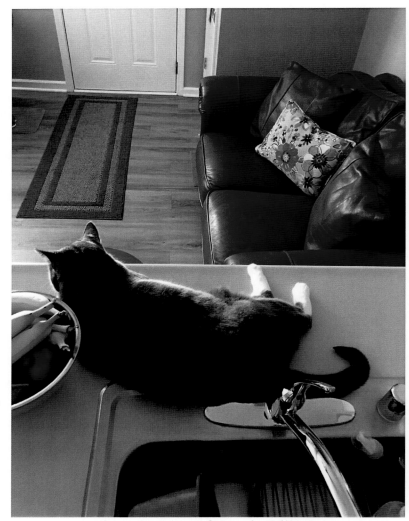

Photo Courtesy of Pamela Willeroy

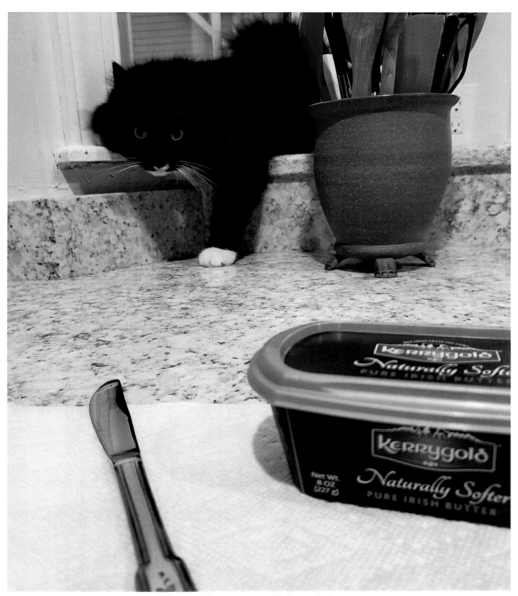

Photo Courtesy of Nora Adams

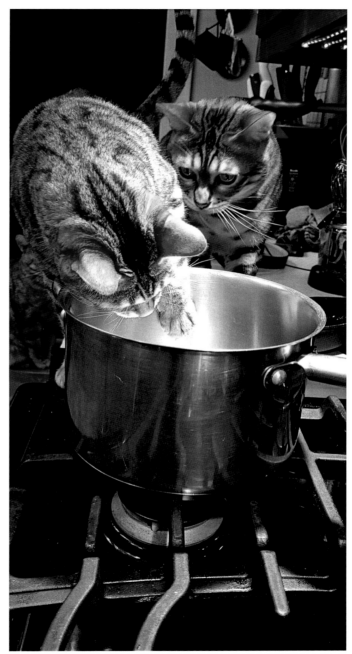

Photo Courtesy of Christopher Robinson

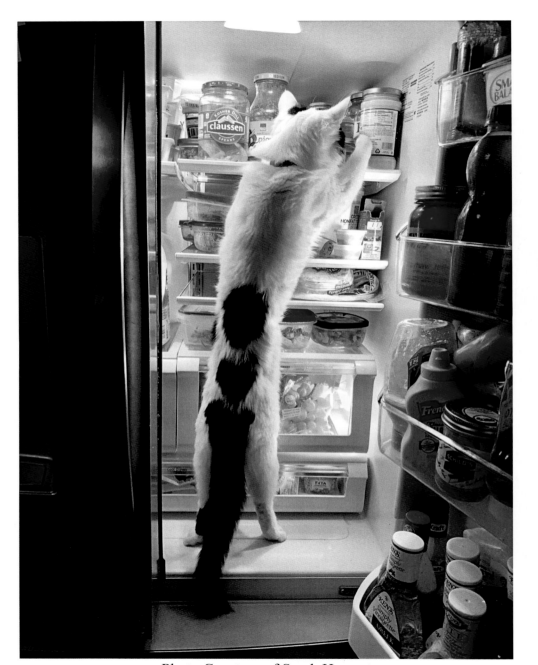

Photo Courtesy of Sarah Harvest

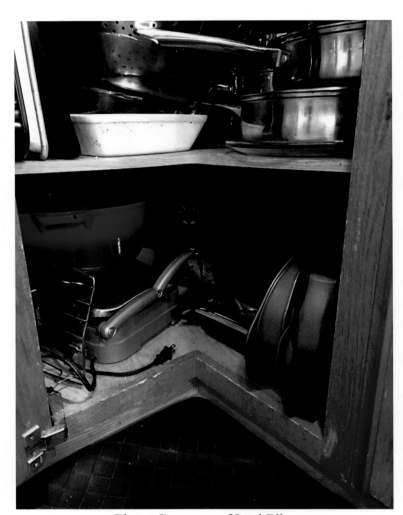

Photo Courtesy of Lori Pike

Nibbles & Bits

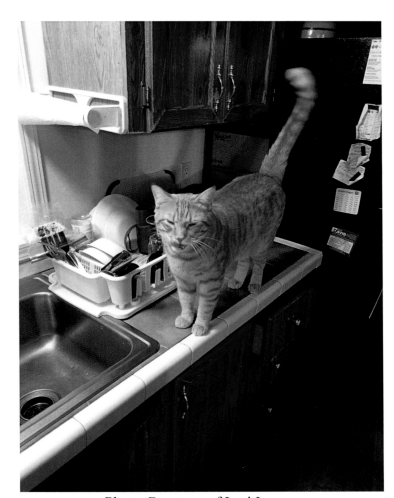

Photo Courtesy of Lari Larson

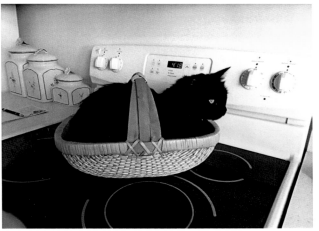

Photo Courtesy of Barbara Biro

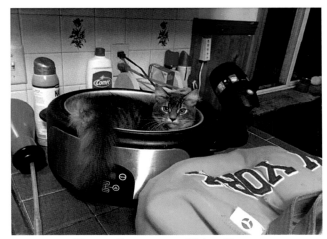

Photo Courtesy of Lisa Reese

Miss Jane's Charleston Cheese Dip

I first heard the legend of Jane from one of our kids who told me that she was pretty much the best cook in the world and that I would really like her because "she has like, a hundred cats." A hundred cats turned out to be more like ten cats, which is still awe-inspiring, and she really is an amazing cook. She moved recently and as fate would have it, her new neighbor rescues cats and seems to have about a dozen or so of the magnificent creatures on hand at all times. What bliss. Anyway, Jane shared this recipe, which comes with a hearty endorsement from her cat, Morticia. As Jane tells it, "one night I had a group of ladies over from our local club. I went to the door to greet the first guests, and when I turned back into the house, there on the dining room table stood Morticia – her whole face submerged in the dip. In one motion I snatched up Morticia with one hand, and the dip with the other. I scraped off the top, added more bacon bits, and my guests knew nothing!" The moral of the story is, bacon fixes everything. And also, if Morticia loves it that much, how can you possibly go wrong?

½ cup mayonnaise
8 oz cream cheese
1 cup sharp cheddar cheese, grated
½ cup Monterey Jack cheese, grated
1 dash cayenne pepper

8 slices bacon, cooked crisp and finely crumbled
8 Ritz crackers, crushed

Optional: 2 green onions, finely chopped

Preheat oven to 350°.

In a medium, bowl, mix the mayonnaise, cream cheese, cheddar, Monterey Jack, cayenne, and green onions, if using. Transfer the mixture to a shallow baking dish.

Top mixture with the cracker crumbs and bake for 15 minutes, or until heated through. Remove from oven and top with the crumbled bacon. Serve immediately with corn chips or crackers. And remember, if necessary, to remove your cat's face from the dish before your guests get a peek.

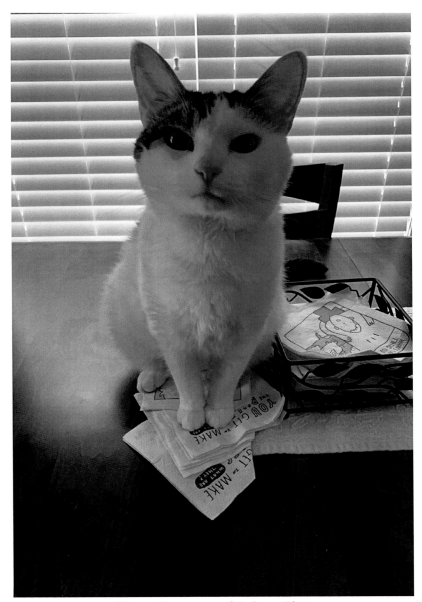

Photo Courtesy of Arlena Titta

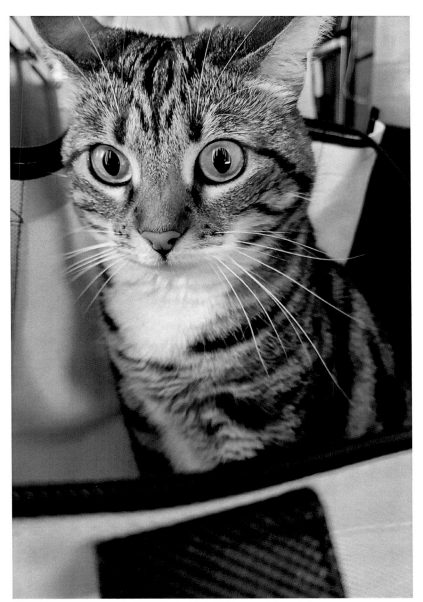

Photo Courtesy of Donald Veith

Spooky LouLou's Mango Salsa

Arizonans know and love their salsa. Jennifer Blackwell makes a mean version that you'd almost rather eat with a spoon than a chip. Jennifer is the kind of cat lady we all aspire to be. She's a radio powerhouse, a professional photographer, a great mom, and has one of the wildest cat stories ever. A story you'd swear inspired Stephen King. When she was a kid, her neighbor had a 10 year-old cat with some serious health issues. The vet gently told the family that Loulou didn't have long. So, when the neighbor found Loulou prostrate in the sun one afternoon, she wept, then got a shovel, and commenced to digging a grave in the rocky desert soil. Imagine her shock when she found Loulou sitting on the front porch the next afternoon, dirt in her ears but otherwise just as pleased with herself as could be. Jennifer says, "We think maybe Loulou had a stroke or some other kind of event? Because the neighbor said she never moved in all the time it took to dig her grave." *Pet Semetary*, anyone? Now, when Jennifer's son, Jace, goes to visit his grandparents, he always suggests that if the neighbor lady sees him napping on the couch, maybe hold off a bit on the burial. Loulou has since passed for real – totally verified this time - but her memory lives on. Someday Jace will be telling his own kids this story, and he'll for sure pass down his mama's salsa recipe.

4 fresh, ripe mangoes, diced
  (aim for 1/8th inch squares)
  OR 1 lb. pre-cut mangoes
1 bundle fresh cilantro

1 medium yellow onion, peeled and finely diced
2 jalapeno peppers, seeded and diced*
¼ tsp salt

*For a milder salsa, use just one jalapeno. Make sure to check the heat scale of your peppers before purchasing. Pepper pungency is measured on something called the Scoville Heat Scale. The higher the Scoville rating, the hotter the pepper. Jalapenos can range from 2,500-10,000 Scoville units! Seeding the pepper will reduce some of the heat – just be careful to wash your hands thoroughly after handling.

Holding the cilantro bundle by the stems, submerge in water for at least 45 seconds. Dry with a clean cloth or paper towel. Remove the larger stems, and, with a sharp knife, finely chop the leaves and remaining stems.

Combine mangoes, onion, cilantro, and jalapeno in a bowl. Add salt. Cover and chill – then enjoy!

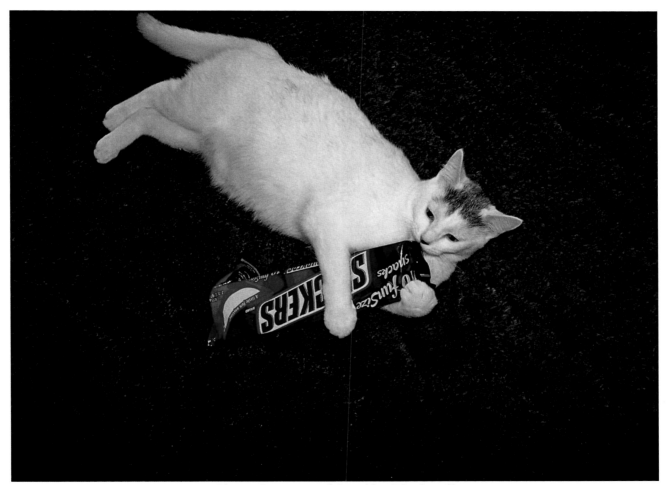
Photo Courtesy of Jennifer Blackwell

Grilled Honey Mint Nectarines with Burrata

Have you ever had burrata? Picture this: tender buffalo-milk mozzarella cheese formed into a pillow stuffed with delicate threads of mozzarella swimming in cream. It's ridiculously decadent. It's meant to be eaten very fresh so if you happen to bump into it, eat it immediately. It's what angels taste like, probably. It's that good, that rich, that otherworldly. It usually doesn't make it to dinner around here because self-control is not possible with burrata. But one day, with too many farmer's market nectarines and a batch of honey mint simple syrup we'd made for mojitos lying around, the burrata managed to make it onto a plate. I've tried this with peaches and plums too – I think you could maybe grill an old oven mitt, drizzle with it with the honey mint and spoon on the burrata and it'd be delicious. Is this a salad? A dessert? Who cares? If you happen to have a loaf of crusty bread, it's a meal.

3 ripe nectarines, halved and pitted
3 burrata balls
2 tbsp olive oil
1 cup honey
1 cup water
1 cup fresh, clean mint leaves, roughly chopped, plus a 6-8 leaves finely julienned

First, make the simple syrup. In a small saucepan, combine honey and water. Bring to a boil, stir well, remove from heat. Place the mint leaves into something heat proof – I use a Pyrex measuring cup. Carefully pour the honey syrup over the mint and set aside for 10-15 minutes. Strain liquid into a clean glass jar and discard the leaves. Once it's completely cooled, refrigerate. It will last a couple of weeks and is great in iced tea, cocktails, etc.

Heat the grill – ours is a gas grill and I set it on medium for this. Brush the cut halves of the fruit with a little oil and place cut side down on the grate. Grill without turning for 5-8 minutes – you just want those beautiful grill marks and for the natural sugars to caramelize a bit. Place each nectarine face-up on a small plate. Drizzle with a bit of the honey mint syrup. Cut each burrata ball carefully in half and spoon the cheese onto the plate next to the grilled fruit. Shower each with a bit of the julienned mint. Even people who are like, "Girl, these cats walking around your kitchen make me sick" will devour this and forget alllllllll about how Princess PuffPuff likes to nap on the cutting board.

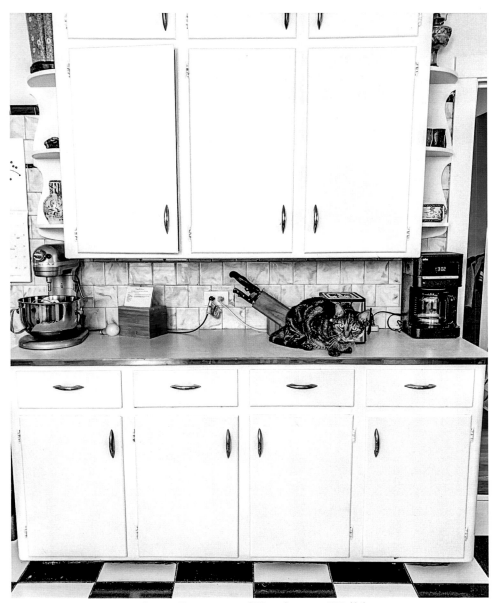

Photo Courtesy of Harrington Weihl

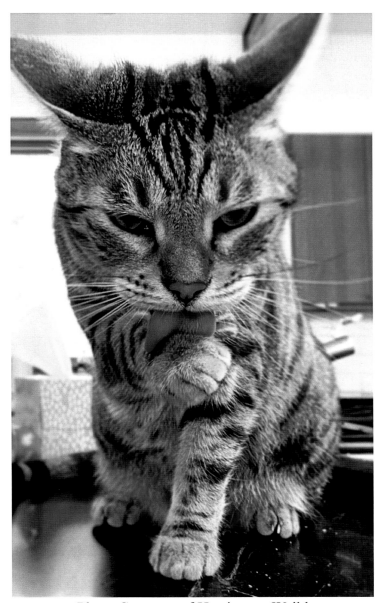

Photo Courtesy of Harrington Weihl

Oven-Baked Buffalo Wings

We went through a hardcore wing phase around here. We'd haul gallons of peanut oil home, fry huge batches of wings, trash the whole kitchen, and be faced with some godawful cleanup. Takeout turned out to be way cheaper and much easier. Then the pandemic hit. When the only chicken we could find at Costco was a jumbo three-pack of wings, it was time to experiment. I borrowed a trick I'd been taught to getting oven-fried chicken crispy: baking powder. The finished wings get a dunk in a bubbling hot sauce, then go back into the oven for a few minutes to tighten everything up. I like Frank's Red Hot sauce for this, but Texas Pete is a close second. This is a super easy recipe to double or triple for a crowd, and any leftovers refrigerate well and are great the next day. You can also make this with full-size drumsticks (aka Godzilla wings), or boneless thighs. In fact, you can just use the seasoning mix and skip the sauce altogether – the chicken is great all by itself.

Warning: even the most civilized cat will try to steal one of these. And when they do, they'll leave a trail of buffalo sauce all over your house. You don't want that. Trust me.

3 lbs. chicken wings
1 tbsp baking powder
2 tsp onion powder
2 tsp garlic powder
½ tsp smoked paprika
½ tsp kosher salt

½ tsp black pepper
1 cup hot sauce of your choice
2 tbsp butter
1 tbsp honey
Celery, carrot sticks, and bleu cheese or ranch dressing

Preheat oven to 425°. Line a large baking sheet with foil and place a wire rack on it.

Thoroughly combine baking powder, onion and garlic powders, paprika, salt, and pepper. Pat wings dry with a paper towel, place in a Ziploc bag, add seasoning mixture and shake till wings are coated. Place wings on wire rack and back for 20 minutes. Turn wings and allow to bake for another 20-25 minutes. Larger wings may take 50-60 minutes to reach an internal temperature of 165°.

Meanwhile, in a small saucepan, heat hot sauce, butter, and honey until just simmering. When wings are fully baked, remove from oven into a large bowl. Pour that bubbling hot sauce over the wings and toss to coat. Return the sauced wings to the wire rack and slide them back into the oven for 5 minutes. Serves 4 as a meal, 8 as an appetizer.

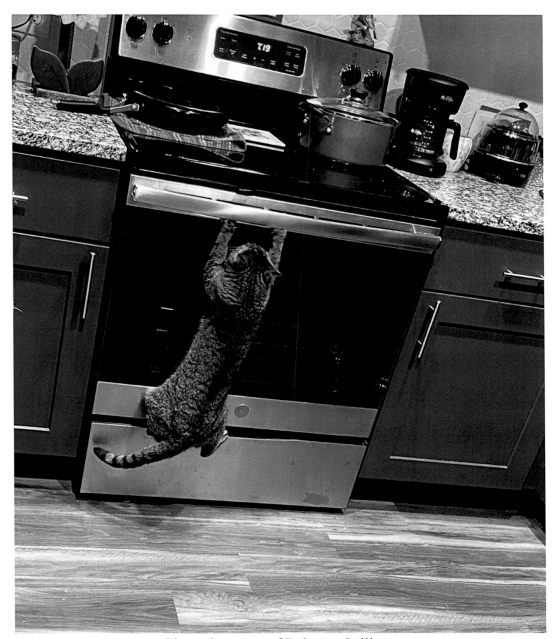

Photo Courtesy of Rebecca Sullivan

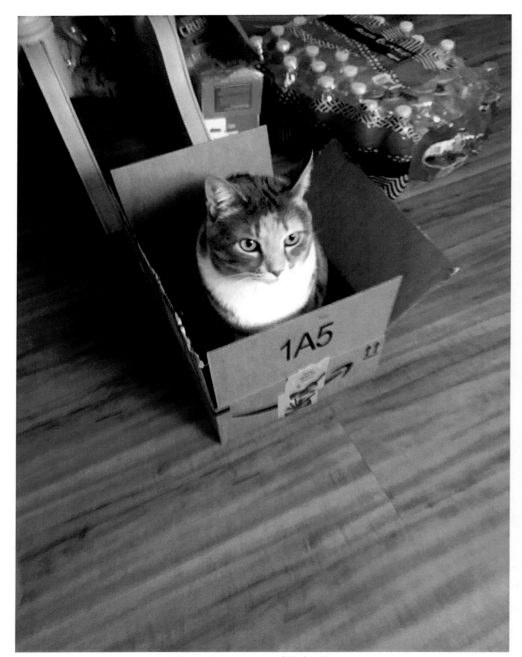

Photo Courtesy of Erin Truett

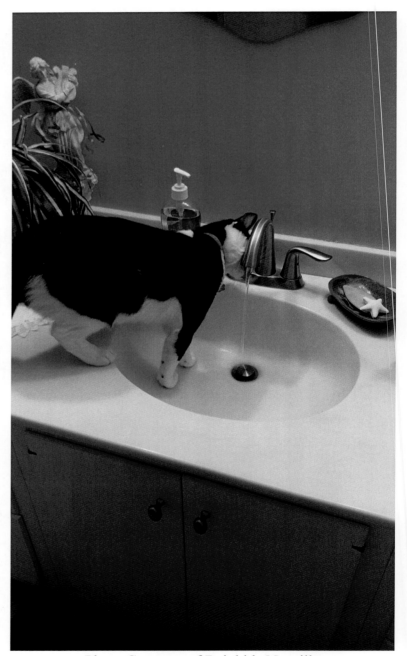

Photo Courtesy of Reinhide Norville

Bake It

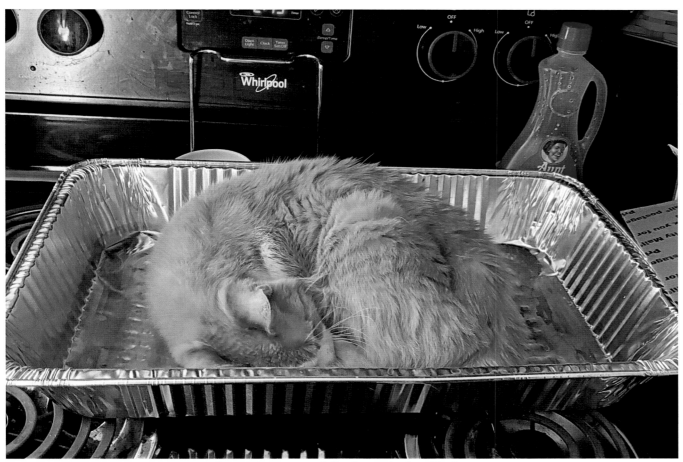

Photo Courtesy of Carlene Taylor-Harlow

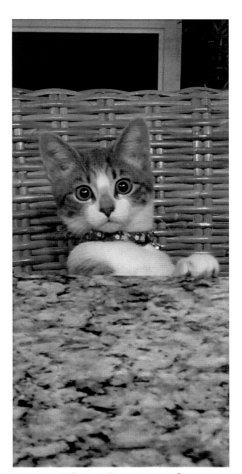

Photo Courtesy of
Melissa McDonnell

Mary Loves Bob Popovers

This is pretty romantic: after their wedding, Mary told Bob she wanted to learn to cook one of his favorite dishes. Considering she'd already brought a magnificent beast of a cat into his life, a cat that insists on sleeping on his pillow (Bob's allergic to cats), and refuses to eat unless Bob stands and watches, offering to make popovers was really above and beyond. Some men are just lucky that way. Speaking of luck, the cat, Kiki, also chose Bob to be her personal litter valet. His reward for the tough work of scooping, sweeping, and watching the cat eat? A huge, tender popover right out of the oven. Yum! Who's the cat daddy king now, Bob?!

4 large eggs (Mary often uses just 3)   1 ½ cups all-purpose flour
1 ½ cups milk   ½ tsp salt
3 tbsp butter, melted

Preheat oven to 450° and position a rack on the lower shelf. The top of the fully risen popovers should be about midway up the height of the oven.

Thoroughly grease a standard 12 cup muffin tin or, better yet, a popover pan.

Whisk together the eggs, milk, and salt until no streaks are showing!

Add the flour all at once and beat with a wire whisk until frothy and there are no clumps. Stir in the melted butter, combining quickly.

Pour the batter into the muffin or popover tin, filling each cup 2/3 full.

Bake the popovers for 20 minutes WITHOUT opening the oven door! Reduce heat to 350° (again, do not open the oven door) and bake for an additional 10-15 minutes until the popovers are a deep, golden brown.

If you plan to serve the popovers immediately – which Mary recommends – remove from oven and poke the tip of a knife into the top pf each popover to release steam and prevent sogginess. Drop a pat of butter into each popover and serve with jam! Or not! Enjoy!

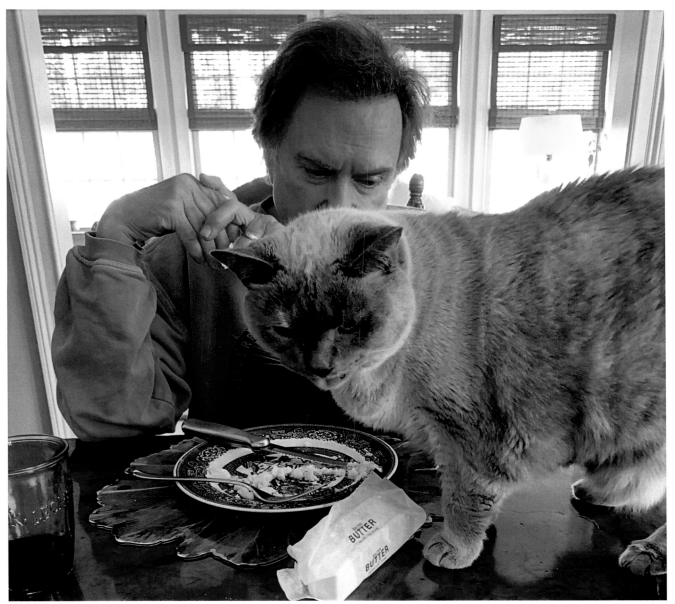

Photo Courtesy of Mary Lacey

Pumpkin Spice Lovers Bread

The great thing about pumpkin bread is that you can pretend it isn't cake as you're eating it for breakfast or in the middle of the night. Plus, pumpkin is a vegetable so look at you being all kinds of virtuous. For this recipe, I amped up the spicy and substituted applesauce for half of the necessary oil, mostly so that I could justify topping it with a buttery, crunchy streusel. (I read once that replacing a cup of oil with a cup of applesauce in your baked goods saves about 1800 calories, so heck yes!) Also, I use ground allspice instead of ground cloves because I love the little peppery kick it has, but if allspice isn't handy, ground cloves are great. These loaves freeze well – and if you slice and wrap each piece individually, you can grab one from the freezer anytime you need a PSL fix or a healthy treat for a school lunch. This is one you'll mix entirely by hand, which is kind of a satisfying experience, especially when the rest of your day is eaten up by technology and gadgets. Plus, it's a fun way to get little kids involved in the kitchen.

1 15 oz can pumpkin puree
1/2 cup unsweetened applesauce
½ cup vegetable oil
4 large eggs
2 ¾ cup brown sugar
½ cup water
1 ½ tsp pure vanilla extract
3 ½ cup all-purpose flour
2 tsp baking soda
1 ½ tsp salt
1 tsp ground nutmeg
1 tsp ground cinnamon
1 tsp ground ginger

1 tsp ground allspice

Streusel topping:

½ cup all-purpose flour
¼ cup rolled oats
¼ cup brown sugar
¼ cup white sugar
5 tbsp butter – to cut into small cubes –
1 ½ tsp cinnamon
1 tsp ground ginger
1 tsp ground nutmeg
Pinch of salt

Preheat oven to 350°.

Grease and flour 2 9x5 loaf pans (I also line the bottom of my pans with parchment paper to make it easier to remove the finished loaves).

In a large bowl, whisk all dry ingredients together until combined: flour, baking soda, salt, and spices.

In a separate large bowl, use a big spoon to gently blend pumpkin, sugar, applesauce, eggs, and vanilla extract. (I like to crack the eggs into a measuring cup and use a fork to just barely beat the yolks and whites together before adding to the pumpkin mixture). Fold in the dry ingredients, stirring until just combined – overworking the batter can make the finished product tough. You'll see how the applesauce already gives the bread a springier texture, anyway, so definitely don't beat the batter to death!

Divide batter evenly between prepared pans.

To make the topping, whisk together the flour, oats, sugars, and spices. Add the cubed butter, using a pastry cutter or a fork to work it in until large or coarse crumbs form. Sprinkle over both loaves, thoroughly covering each.

Bake for 50-60 minutes. Test for doneness at the :50 mark. Loaves are ready when a skewer or toothpick inserted in the center comes out clean. Cool in pans for 10 minutes. Then, instead of inverting onto a wire rack finish cooling (you don't want to lose a crumb of that topping), carefully slide a large metal spatula around the rim of the pan, then underneath the loaf to gently dislodge it. Yields 2 loaves.

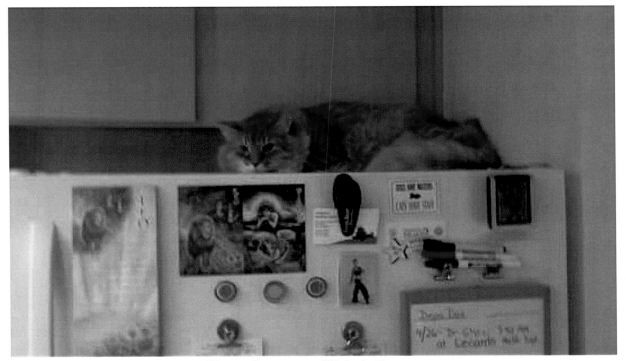

Photo Courtesy of Valerie Brown

Joni & Nick's Cathead Biscuits

I thought that cathead biscuits were shaped like, well, a cat's head. Tragically, I now know that they got the name for their size; not for having ears or whiskers. Luckily, one of my most favorite people has an authentic recipe for catheads that she's happy to share. Joni Eargle Nash Case is smart and kind – a fantastic Southern cook – and someone everyone knows they can count on in a crisis, no matter how big or small. When Joni was a little girl, her grandmother had a big, mean old calico cat named Tilley. Tilley's only love was for Nanny. Everyone else got a baleful glare accompanied by hissing and spitting. As Nanny was getting up in years, it was decided that she needed to hire some help. Showing the new housekeeper around, Tilley followed, hissing, from room to room, keeping what Joni called a hateful distance. The poor woman kept tiptoeing past the spitting beast until finally, having not spotted a litter box, she ventured a hesitant, "Mrs. Eargle? Does your cat go outdoors?" The answer was a firm no. Tilley never left the house. The housekeeper pondered this for a moment then tried again. "She never goes outside?" No, came the answer. Never. Puzzled and unable to contain herself, she finally asked, "But, then, where does she…step aside?" In my whole life I don't believe I've ever encountered a more polite, genteel euphemism. And for the record, Tilley stepped aside down in the basement. Tilley's tale got us on the subject of cathead biscuits, which Joni's old friend Nick, a real Cat Daddy himself, showed her how to make 35 years ago, using this recipe. (The handwritten original is a masterpiece of minimalism – great home cooks just know what they're doing but dang, it can be a tough act to follow.)

3 cups self-rising flour, plus more for kneading and rolling
1 cup vegetable shortening

1 ¾ cup milk, approximately (you really do have to feel your way through this one)
OPTIONAL: 2 tbsp melted butter

Preheat oven to 450°.

In a large bowl, combine flour and shortening. Cut together with a pastry blender (or hand mixer, which Nick suggests – maybe you have one in the back of a drawer?) Moisten with a bit of milk, and stir, adding more milk if needed until the dough is holding together with a sticky consistency.

Mound flour generously on your work surface. Turn out the dough, sprinkling more flour on top. Knead the dough with the palm of your hand, turning the dough and folding it. Do this 4-6 times, then pat and flatten the dough with your hands until it is a smooth disk about 2 inches thick. Dip a 3 ½ inch round cutter in flour and cut your biscuits. Place on an ungreased sheet. (Tip: for tender biscuits, snuggle them up close. For crispier, spread them out on the pan so that their sides won't touch as they bake.) Be careful not to overwork the dough as you cut, because you want the end result to be fluffy and tender. Be gentle with your biscuit dough!

Prick tops of cut biscuits and if you like, brush with the melted butter. Bake for 25 minutes, or until both tops and bottoms are a nice golden brown. Transfer to a wire rack for a brief cooling, then serve warm. Yields 10 biscuits, each the size of a cat's head.

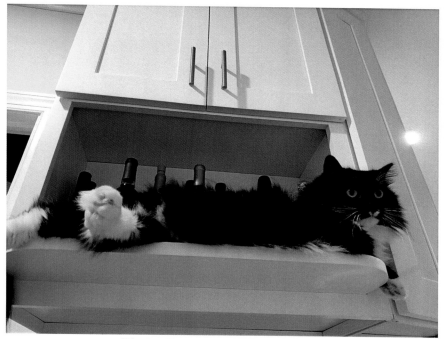

Photo Courtesy of Nora Adams

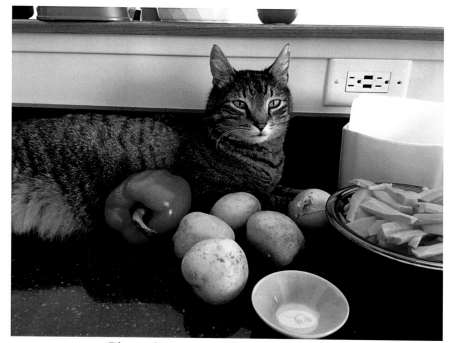

Photo Courtesy of Suzanne Hazelton

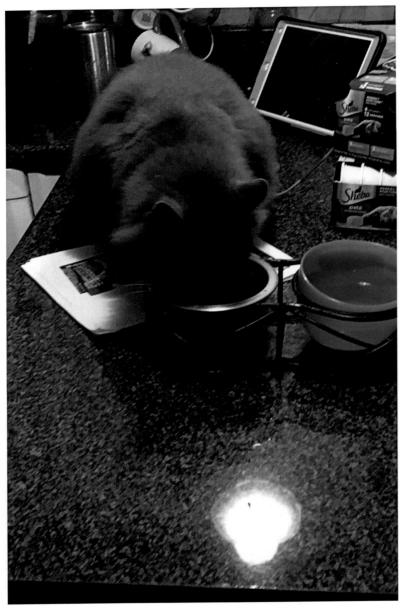

Photo Courtesy of Sarah Gibson

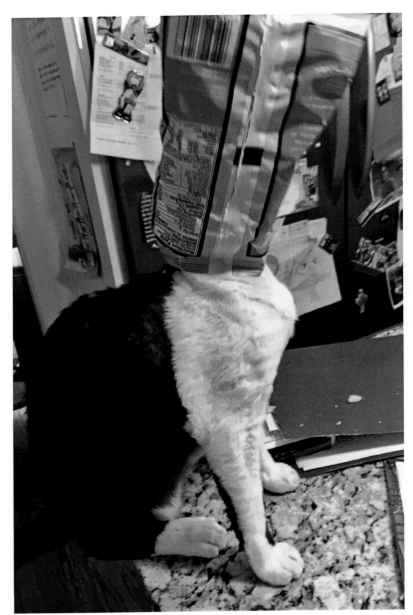

Photo Courtesy of Sheri Lynch

Serve It On The Side

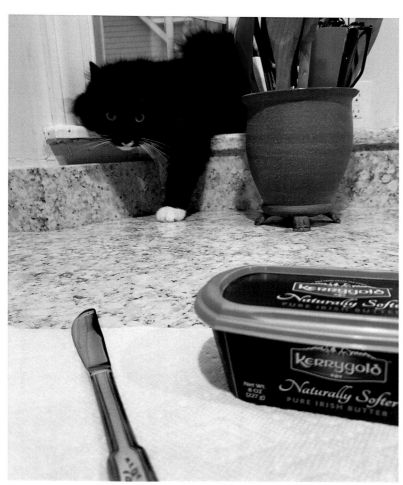

Photo Courtesy of Nora Adams

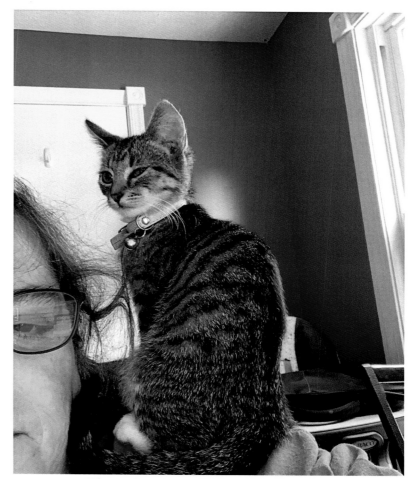

Photo Courtesy of Meredith Chandler

Hot German Potato Salad Lambeau

This comes from one of my most favorite cat lady queens, Anne Oberlander: "My cat, Lambeau, a gorgeous Ragdoll, is named after the finest sporting venue in the land: Lambeau Field, in Green Bay, WI. As native Wisconsinites, my husband and I are, of course, Packer fans. Those who hail from the Dairy State are born this way. Packer fandom is a reflex, an instinct. We've been lucky enough to attend several games at Lambeau Field, where the tailgating tradition is fully, heartily embraced. Any tailgate gathering is bound to feature our native foods. We Badgers, many of us of German descent, love our bratwurst grilled, our beer cold, and our potato salad hot. This recipe involves what we consider our four major food groups: bacon, potatoes, cheese, and Other Things. No cheese in this recipe, but you can always serve slices on the side. This is a version of the classic recipe in *The Joy of Cooking* by Irma Rombauer, which my mother referred to reverently only as The Rombauer."

6 medium-size redskin potatoes, unpeeled
4 strips bacon – or 5 or 6 n- chopped
¼ cup chopped onion
¼ cup chopped celery
1 large dill pickle, chopped
¼ cup water or stock

½ cup apple cider vinegar
1 tsp sugar
½ tsp salt
¼ tsp dry mustard
¼ tsp celery seed
1 tsp cornstarch

Cook the potatoes in a covered saucepan until fork tender. Don't overcook! Drain in a colander and rinse briefly in cold water. Peel and slice while still warm. Set aside.

In a heated skillet, sauté the chopped bacon until brown and crispy. Using a slotted spoon, remove the bacon and set aside. Reserve the drippings. Sauté the onion and celery in the bacon drippings until golden. Stir in the dill pickle.

Add the water, vinegar, sugar, salt, dry mustard, and celery seed to the skillet, stirring to combine. Sprinkle the cornstarch over top and stir in. Bring the mixture, stirring, until slightly thickened.

Gently fold the potato slices and bacon bits into the skillet. Serve hot. Serves 4-6.

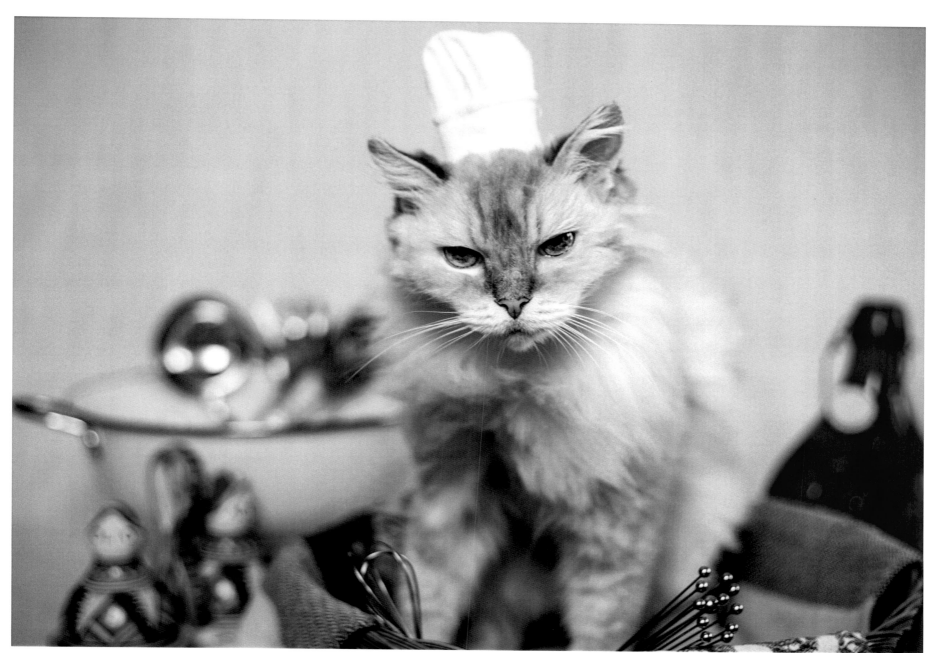
Photo Courtesy of Anne Oberlander

Skillet Sweet Corn and Bacon

The phrase "meatless meal" means something different to my husband than it does for me. I discovered this when he poked sadly around in a bowl of black beans and rice and asked, "No bacon? No fatback? No streak o' lean?" Okay, first of all, fatback and streak o' lean were things I'd read about in books, but never actually cooked with or eaten, and second, who wants to tell him that any kind of pork is still, well, meat? The thing is, cooking veggies with pork is not only a classic Southern technique, it's absolutely delicious. It's just not "meatless" no matter how much he wants to argue. One day when I was playing around with a version of homemade creamed corn, he suggested leaving out the cream. Which basically left a skillet full of sweet corn and bacon. Which turned out to be super tasty – so much so that most of it was eaten before it could even make it to the table. Fresh corn or frozen corn both work – you could probably use canned corn as long as you drain it. Now that I think about it, it would actually be downright merciful to treat canned corn this way.

4 ears sweet corn, shucked, kernels removed
(OR 3 cups frozen corn kernels, thawed and drained
OR 3 cups canned corn, drained)
4-6 slices bacon, chopped into 1-inch pieces

¼ cup green onions sliced, plus 1 tbsp reserved
1 tsp sugar
1 ½ tsp kosher salt
Freshly ground black pepper to taste

Heat a skillet – cast iron if you have one – over medium-high heat. Cook bacon, watching carefully and turning occasionally, until crisp. Remove bacon to a paper towel-lined plate to drain. Reserve at least 3 tbsp bacon grease and pour off the rest.

Add corn and reserved bacon drippings to pan, along with green onion, sugar, salt, and pepper. Sauté, stirring frequently, for 5 minutes. Stir in reserved bacon. Taste to adjust salt and pepper. Top with reserved green onions. Serves 4 – unless you've managed to eat most of it with a large spoon directly from the pan, in which case, good luck to anyone not lucky enough to be in the kitchen with you.

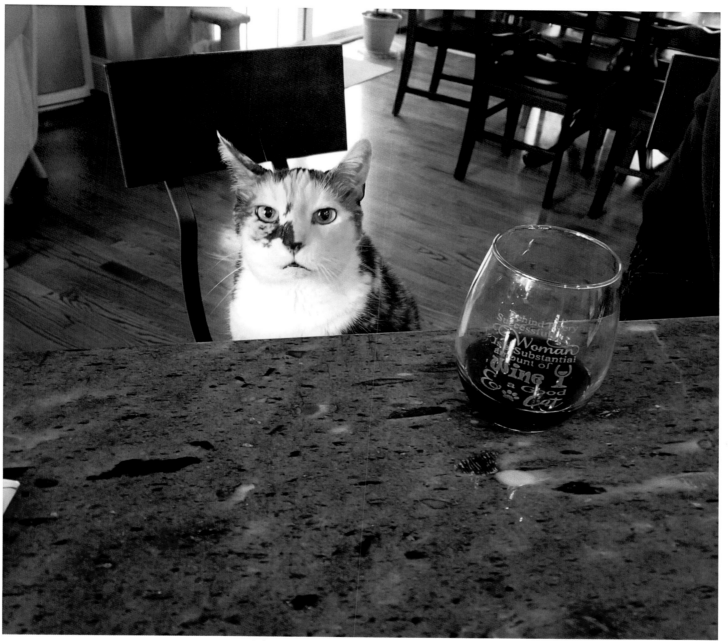
Photo Courtesy of Jennifer Salley

Jack Henry's Breakfast Potatoes

Jack Henry is a cat who knows what he likes, and how to get his human to make it. His human is Courtney Armstrong, a woman of so many dazzling talents that it's almost unfair. A gifted designer and seamstress, Courtney can whip up a one-of-a-kind fairy costume or a queenly headdress or a sassy elf suit out of things you might happen to have stashed around the house.

But how is her cat Jack Henry so good at getting his way? It all began when he was the scrawny, grey runt of the litter in a box of kittens at the vet's office. Courtney's mom thought she wanted the lone orange kitten in the bunch, but Jack Henry stretched out one skinny paw, tapped her on the arm, and meowed. !2 years later, Courtney reports that he's still the same sweet, noisy boy who doesn't hesitate to reach out and use his paws and his voice to get your attention. He was utterly devoted to her mom while she lived, and now loyally watches over Courtney – and whatever she happens to be eating. Like these potatoes, which are super easy to make and will impress your human guests no end.

4 baking potatoes, sliced into bite-sized pieces*

6-8 cloves garlic, peeled, crushed, chopped

1 large onion, peel & quarter, then slice quarters into thirds

½ cup olive oil

Salt & pepper

Optional add-ins:

1 cup cherry tomatoes, halved

1 bell pepper, cored, seeded, and sliced

6 strips bacon, cooked crisp and crumbled

Optional seasoning:

1 tsp dried thyme OR dill OR lemon pepper OR Old Bay

1 tsp garlic powder – (for those who just really, really like garlic

*Jack Henry's No Opposable Thumbs Potato Trick: slice each potato in half lengthwise. Slice the halves again. Chop each quarter into 3 bite-size pieces.

Preheat oven to 400°. Line a baking sheet with aluminum foil (for easier cleanup).

Spread onion slices in a single layer on baking sheet; season with a sprinkle of salt and pepper. (If adding bell pepper OR bacon, add these to the layer of onions.)

Layer potatoes over onion. Sprinkle fresh garlic over the potato layer. Pour olive oil over the pan and give the potatoes a gentle stir. Season again with salt and pepper – and any additional optional seasoning of your choice.

Back for 20-25 minutes. Flip the potatoes and sprinkle lightly with salt and pepper. Layer cherry tomatoes over top, if using. Bake for another 20- minutes.

Serves 6. Any leftovers will keep well in the refrigerator and can be reheated in the microwave.

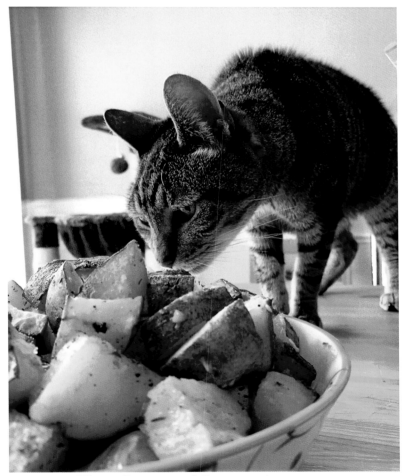

Photo Courtesy of Courtney Armstrong

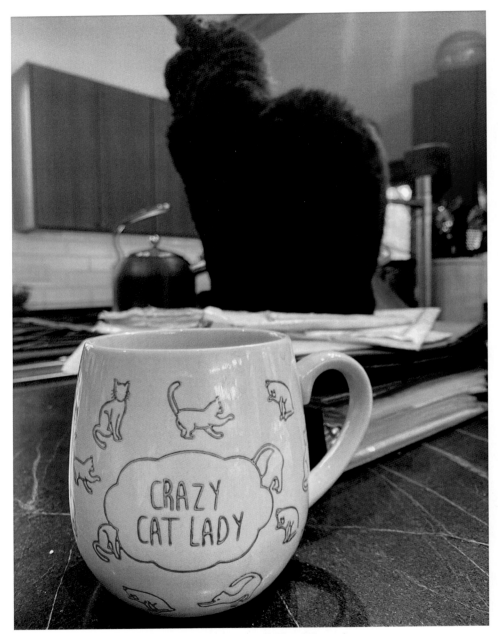

Photo Courtesy of Sheri Lynch

Mains

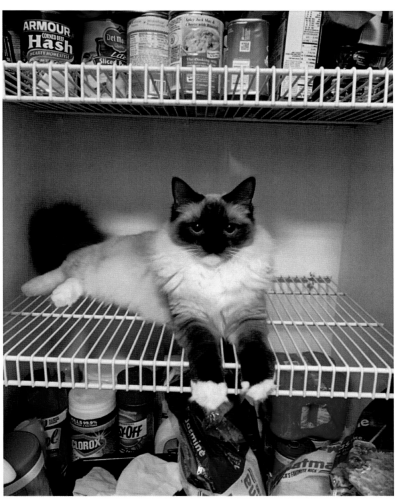

Photo Courtesy of Crystal Allen

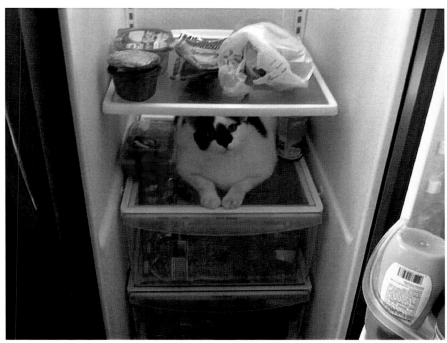

Photo Courtesy of Melissa Chanault

(Not Exactly) Nana Sarah's Fried Chicken Tenders

A Southern man's reverence for his mama and her cooking is something I'd only read about in books – then I married one and discovered that, yes, ain't nothing ever, ever gonna be better than his mama's version. Sadly, Nana Sarah passed away suddenly and unexpectedly, taking her utterly divine fried chicken recipe and technique with her. Meanwhile, I'd never fried a piece of chicken in my life. After much experimenting, I landed on this. Now you know it's not his mama's – especially since I fry it in a big Dutch oven, not a cast iron skillet. This is, of course, pure heresy. Heresy or not, frying in a Dutch oven limits oil splatters, which makes cleanup easier. Authentic or not, it's crunchy and delicious and awesome the next day, ice cold right out of the fridge.

2 lbs. boneless skinless chicken tenders
1 cup all-purpose flour
1 cup panko breadcrumbs
1 ½ tbsp onion powder
1 ½ tbsp garlic powder
¾ tsp chili powder

½ tsp smoked paprika
1 tsp salt
1 tsp freshly ground black pepper
3 large eggs
1 ½ cup peanut or canola oil

(Note: if you're feeling ambitious, you might marinate the chicken in buttermilk with a couple of shots of Tabasco. Just pop it all in a bowl or Ziploc bag and leave it in the fridge for a few hours.)

Heat the oil in your Dutch oven to 375° – it's important to not let the oil get too hot! Test the temperature with your thermometer once the oil begins to shimmer.

Next, preheat oven to 250°, and lay a wire rack over a baking sheet.

In a large shallow bowl, combine flour, panko, and seasonings. If it seems overly seasoned, don't worry. It needs to be, promise. In a separate shallow bowl, lightly beat the eggs with a fork.

Dip each tender first into the egg wash, then into the seasoned flour and panko. Make sure each piece is thoroughly coated. Fry the tenders in batches of 3 (or 4, if they're on the smaller side). You never want to crowd the pan, or the temp of the oil will drop, and your tenders will be soggy and greasy instead of light and crunchy. Fry for 4-5 minutes, then turn and fry another 4-5. I test them with an instant-read thermometer to be sure of doneness (you want an internal temp of 165°). Place cooked tenders on the prepared wire rack and leave in oven as you cook the rest of the chicken. This will keep it warm and crisp till you're ready to serve. And speaking of, this serves 6 – unless you have no sides and a huge appetite in which case, serves 4.

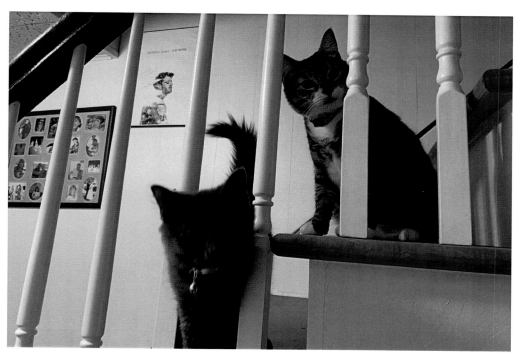
Photo Courtesy of Bonnie Bee

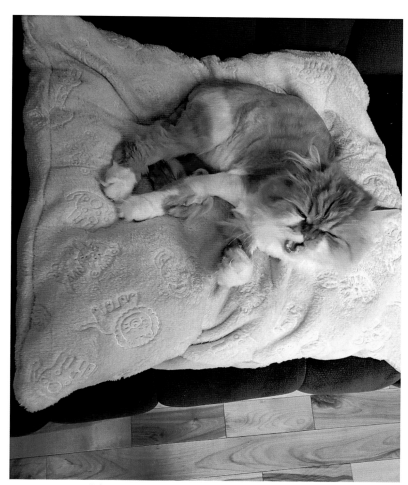
Photo Courtesy of Nicole Gaumond

Grandmom Bartholetti's Meatballs

When I was little, we alternated Sunday dinners between my Grandmom Bartholetti's row home in South Philadelphia and my Grandmom Blackhair's suburban Cape Cod in South Jersey. Pasta was called macaroni, sauce was called gravy, and meatballs were at the center of a bitter feud. Whose were better? Whose did we love best? I was fiercely loyal to Blackhair in all things but one: Bartholetti's meatballs were better. Not just better, but next-level velvety and incredible. It took me a long time to pry the recipe out of my mom's hands, and when I finally got it and learned it contained milk (I'm allergic), I was forced to come up with a hybrid version that borrowed from both of my battling grandmothers. It's mostly Bartholetti's recipe though. And even though we moved out west when I was 7 and didn't have her meatballs again until I was all grown up, I know she'd be pleased to have won the fight.

1 lb. lean ground beef

1 lb. ground pork

2 cloves fresh minced garlic

4 eggs, lightly beaten

½ cup plain breadcrumbs

½ cup freshly grated Pecorino Romano cheese

½ cup fresh parsley, finely chopped

½ cup beef broth (or milk, if you prefer)

1 tsp salt

1 tsp freshly ground black pepper

1 tbsp dried basil

Olive oil for browning

Soak the breadcrumbs in the broth (or milk). Take off your jewelry, roll up your sleeves, and wash your hands because the only way to really make a proper meatball is to do it by hand. Place all of the ingredients into a large bowl and very gently combine. The more you work ground meat, the tougher it will be, so the goal here is to handle the meat as little as possible. Carefully roll the meat into balls – I like to go with something about the size of a lime.

Heat a large Dutch oven over medium. Add about ¼ inch olive oil to the pan and allow to heat for a minute or two. Add meatballs, careful not to crowd the pan – you'll brown them in batches.

IF ADDING TO GRAVY: Fry until a nice golden brown, approximately 2-3 minutes per side. Remove and place on a paper-towel covered plate to drain. When finished, reserve the pan drippings because we'll use those to build the gravy – next recipe. At this stage the meatballs are not cooked all the way through, and will finish in the gravy in a nice, long simmer.

If you just want to eat them up plain or with a jarred sauce (no judgment because life is hard enough), then be sure to cook the meatballs all the way through, about 15 minutes, turning often.

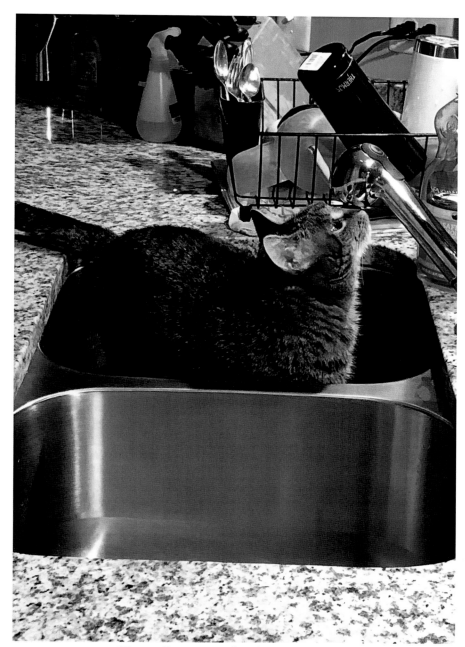

Photo Courtesy of Rebecca Sullivan

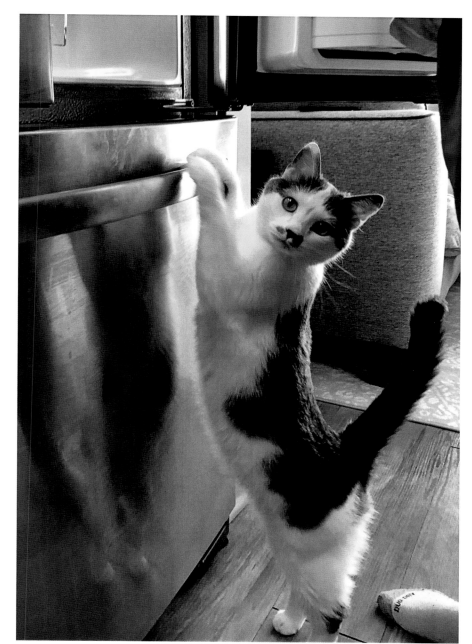

Photo Courtesy of Jill Miracle

Sunday Meatballs and Gravy

In most parts of the world, gravy is brown and, if you're unlucky, lumpy and weird. For lots of Italian American families, 'gravy' is what the rest of the world calls 'spaghetti sauce'. Sunday gravy takes all day to simmer and is as much about the meat as it as about the tomatoes. But why call it gravy? It's a good question. The Italian word for a meat-based sauce is 'ragu', which sounds nothing like 'gravy'. For my relatives, 'ragu" was an abomination in a jar that no self-respecting Italian would eat, but that can't possibly account for the hijacking of the word 'gravy' because other families are less insane. If you really want to be authentic, you'll brown up a pound of Italian sausages along with a pound of pork ribs and toss those into the pot with the meatballs. It's a meatpalooza but you'll die happy.

3 28 oz cans whole peeled San Marzano tomatoes

1 6 oz can tomato paste

6 cloves finely chopped garlic

I small onion, finely chopped

2 cups water OR beef broth*

1 cup dry red wine

2 bay leaves

1 tbsp dried oregano

1 cup fresh basil leaves – sliced into fine ribbons aka julienned

Salt & pepper to taste

Splash of olive oil

One batch lightly browned meatballs
 (see recipe for Grandmom Bartholetti's Meatballs)

Freshly grated Pecorino Romano cheese for serving

Optional: 1 lb. Italian sausage links

1 lb. pork ribs (country or spareribs both work)

Into the pan drippings from your meatball-making experience, lightly brown the sausage. Remove and set aside. Repeat with the pork ribs. (Add another splash of olive oil if needed.)

Now add onions and garlic to the pan, cooking over medium heat just until the onions soften and become translucent. Watch the heat and don't burn the garlic! Carefully pour in the wine and scraping up all those yummy browned bits off the bottom of the pan, cook for about 5 minutes.

Using your hands, crush and break up the San Marzano tomatoes. This is messy, so either wear an apron or don't wear a white shirt. Just reach into the can, grab a handful of tomato and squeeze and crush it right over the pot, pouring any juices that remain in the can into the pot as well. Add tomato paste, water/broth, oregano, basil, bay leaves, and a few grinds of black pepper. Next, carefully sink the ribs, sausages, and meatballs into the tomato mixture.

Bring to a boil, stir, then reduce heat to low. Simmer for 4-6 hours, stirring occasionally to keep meats from sticking to bottom of pan. Just keep an eye on the heat – you want a simmer, not a boil. If gravy thickens too rapidly, you can add a bit more water or broth.

Cook pasta according to package directions. (My favorite pasta for gravy is paccheri, which is like a more substantial penne. Bucatini is also fun – it's a thick, hollow spaghetti.) Pile the meats onto a platter and the pasta and gravy into a large serving bowl. Pass the grated Pecorino Romano, pour a glass of wine, and pretend you're in the Mafia. Now eat! Eat some more!

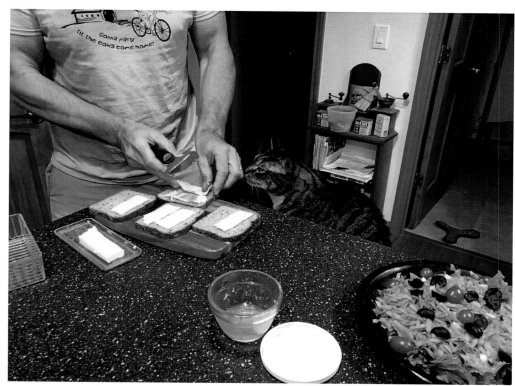

Photo Courtesy of Sue Priest

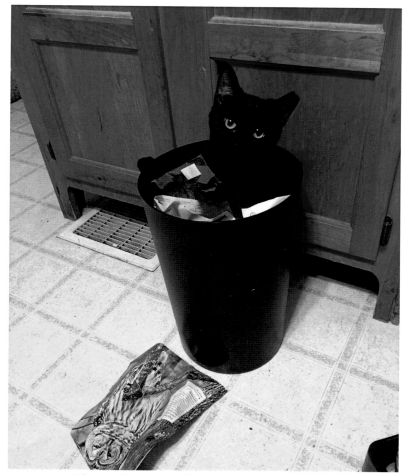

Photo Courtesy of Penny Saskia Kramer

Hot Damn Pork Tenderloin

You know how sometimes you'll buy a little jar of something at the grocery store just out of curiosity? No? Just me then. That's how I first discovered harissa. Harissa is a chili pepper paste that hails from Tunisia. It's so good – lots of heat, but super versatile. It pairs really well with citrus and sweet flavors and can absolutely transform plain old chicken and, in this case, pork tenderloin. Pork tenderloin is lean and not wildly flavorful on its own. But it stands up to a long marinade – 4-24 hours, grills up fast, and when you catch a sale, is a pretty affordable protein that makes for an easy meal, simple or fancy. I almost always butterfly the tenderloin before marinating – the flavors hit more surface area that way. Plus, it'll cook a bit faster and make it easier to avoid overcooking the meat. Use an instant-read thermometer and aim for 145-150 degrees and let the meat rest for a few minutes before slicing. Yes, all of our moms were terrified of trichinosis, so they cooked pork slam to death, but times have changed, and I promise, 150 degrees means it's done. You'll love how juicy and tender the pork is and you'll live.

2 lb. pork tenderloin
½ cup maple syrup
2 tbsp harissa

½ tsp ground cumin
½ tsp garlic powder

Combine syrup, harissa, cumin, and garlic powder. Using the tip of a sharp knife, carefully slide the blade under the silver skin on the tenderloin and peel it away. Butterfly the tenderloin. Make sure the meat is thoroughly coated with the marinade and pop it into the fridge. Dish, container, Ziploc bag – your choice. Just wrap or seal it tightly. Marinate for a minimum of 4 hours, or, even better, overnight.

Remove the meat from the refrigerator at least 30 minutes before grilling. (Don't toss the excess marinade just yet.) If you're using a gas grill, heat one side to High, and leave the other side unlit. Sear the tenderloin for about 7 minutes, then flip it and sear the other side for 5-7 minutes. Using your instant-read thermometer, check the internal temperature. If it reads 145, take it off the grill, make a loose little aluminum foil tent for it, and allow it to rest for a bit – 10 minutes is plenty. If the meat needs a bit of additional cook time, move it to the unlit side of the grill so that it doesn't get too charred, and let that residual heat finish it off.

If you like, pour the remaining marinade into a small saucepan and bring it to a boil. (I do this right on the grill as I'm cooking the pork.) Drizzle this sauce over the meat or whatever starch you serve alongside or even over steamed broccoli. Warning: this will add a real kick of heat to the finished dish, so be careful of overdoing the spicy for eaters who prefer a tamer meal.

Slice. Serves 6.

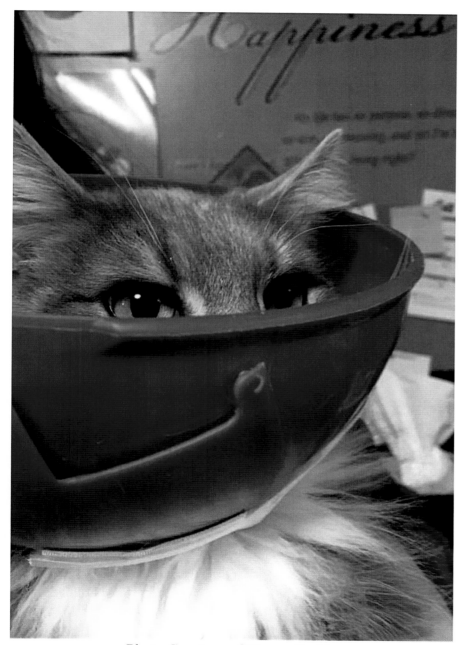

Photo Courtesy of Steven Boddy

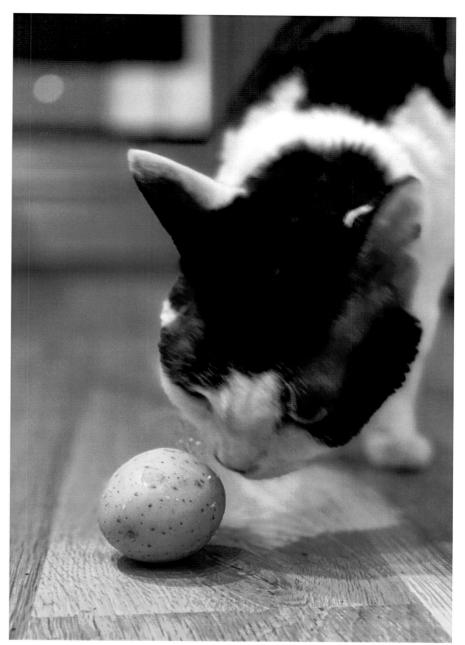

Photo Courtesy of Sheri Lynch

Linguini with White Clam Sauce

This is one of those dishes that seems difficult and special occasion-y but it's actually simple, quick, and made up of ingredients that are easily stocked in your pantry. Keep this stuff on hand and you've got dinner without making a trip to the store. The only fresh ingredients are parsley and lemon zest and honestly, if you're snowed in or just feeling lazy and only have dried parsley, so what? It'll do. No lemon either? Okay, that's sad but not the end of the world. The secret ingredient here is one of my favorite stealth tricks: anchovies. Don't scream in horror. The anchovies melt away leaving only a rich, savory flavor that makes everything better. I sneak them into all sorts of things, from pastas, to soups, to shrimp and grits. Just try it and see.

(And yes, you can absolutely make this with fresh clams and homemade pasta and if you do, please invite me. This is not that recipe. This is more of a bad-weather-feeling lazy-but want-something-delicious situation.)

1 2 oz. tin flat anchovies in olive oil	Zest of ½ lemon (approx. 1 tsp)
4 8 oz. cans chopped or minced clams (reserve liquid!)	Splash of white wine* (approx. 2 tbsp)
¼ cup extra-virgin olive oil	Handful fresh chopped parsley – about ¾ cup OR 4 tbsp dried parsley
1 small onion, finely diced	
4 cloves garlic, finely chopped	1 lb. linguini, prepared according to package instructions,
¼ tsp red pepper flakes	reserve ¼ cup pasta liquid**

In a large, deep skillet over medium heat, sauté the anchovies, using a wooden spoon to break them up until they melt. Add the onion and garlic, stirring frequently until the onions soften. Add the red pepper flakes, reserved clam liquid, wine, and ¼ cup reserved pasta liquid. Stir and allow to simmer for 10-15 minutes. Add clams, parsley, lemon zest. Stir, and cook for another five minutes. Add cooked pasta to pan, tossing thoroughly. Serves 4-6.

*I'm not a white wine drinker, so any time a bottle shows up around here, I freeze any leftovers in snack-size baggies. It stays slushy so it's easy to measure out. You can also skip the wine altogether if you like. It won't be a tragedy. Replace it with either chicken broth, or a 1 tbsp lemon juice and 1 tbsp water.)

**This is the one time where I don't recommend aggressively salting your pasta water while cooking. The anchovy and clams should add enough salt to the dish.

***OPTIONAL: Sometimes I'll add a small can of diced tomatoes (14.5 oz) just because I like the added sweetness and color. It makes my ancestors spin in their graves, but then again, so did my three marriages. Try it and see how you like it. The tomatoes, I mean. Not the marriages.

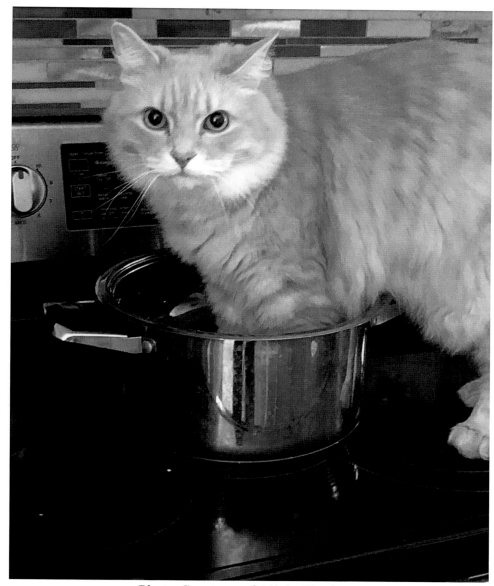

Photo Courtesy of Alicia Charletta

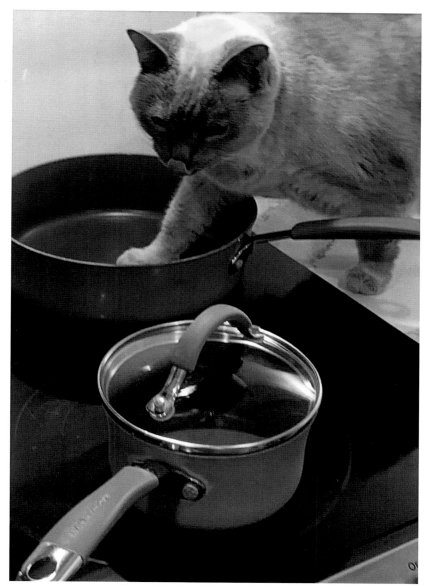

Photo Courtesy of Mary Lacey

Chicken Pie

When I was a kid I thought pot pie was the worst kind of lie: flaky, golden pie crust luring you in only to trap you in a pond of goo in which a single green pea, a Chernobyl-orange cube of carrot, and a miniscule shred of what you sincerely prayed was actually chicken were suspended. Ewww no thanks. Naturally I went on to marry a man who loves it. Because I love pie and chicken and well, him, I decided to try making my own goo-free version. Every time I prepare this recipe, it gets a little tweak. Sometimes I make the crust from scratch, sometimes I use store-bought pie dough. Sometimes I roast a chicken just to make a pie, sometimes I grab a cooked rotisserie chicken from the supermarket. The one constant is a whole lot of chicken. You can actually hoist a slab of this and eat it with your hands. That's how much chicken we're going to stuff into this pie. Also, you can play with the ratio of vegetables. My family hates cooked carrots and won't touch a mushroom, but yours may love those things. Warning: this will have the cats swarming, so you must be fast on your feet with eyes in the back of your head or those little scavengers will snatch that bird right out of your hands.

4 cups roasted chicken, generous-sized shreds	¼ tsp turmeric
1/3 cup carrots, finely diced	2 tbsp fresh parsley, finely chopped
1 cup onion, finely chopped	2 tbsp white wine (optional)
1 cup celery, thinly sliced	¼ cup half-and-half OR heavy cream if you happen to have it
3-4 cups chicken stock	1 egg yolk plus ¼ tsp water
4-6 tbsp unsalted butter*	Kosher salt
¼ cup all-purpose flour	Freshly ground black pepper
¼ tsp dried thyme	1 top & 1 bottom pie crust**

*NOTE: if you've roasted your own chicken, pour the pan drippings into a measuring cup. When the fat separates, spoon out 2 tbsp. You'll use this, along with 4 tbsp butter. Otherwise, use 6 tbsp butter.

**NOTE: I always pre-bake the bottom crust because a soggy pie crust is nasty. It's not hard to do and while it adds an extra step, the results are worth it.

Preheat oven to 375°.

Place a large, deep skillet over medium-high heat, melt the butter (and pan drippings if using). Sauté carrots, onion, and celery until onions soften and become translucent – about 5 minutes. Add the chicken, stir. Evenly sprinkle flour over the contents of the pan; stir to combine. (You're making a fast, rough and tumble roux, and a roux is just flour and fat on its way to becoming sauce or gravy.) Keep stirring for 5 minutes. Pour in 3 cups chicken stock and add the optional white wine. Simmer for 15-20 minutes, stirring occasionally and scraping up the browned bits from the bottom of the pan as you go. As the mixture thickens, add the thyme, turmeric, and a grind of black pepper. Pour in the half-and-half or cream and add the fresh parsley. Stir and allow to cook for just a few minutes more. If it's too thick, splash in a bit more chicken stock. Taste, and add a pinch or two of kosher salt if needed. Remove from heat.

Spoon mixture onto the pre-baked bottom crust. Lay the other crust on top, pressing and crimping the edges to seal. Brush with the egg yolk-water wash. Sprinkle with kosher salt and fresh black pepper. Using a sharp paring knife, cut 4 small slits into the top crust and bake for 30-35 minutes. Let it rest for a few minutes once it comes out of the oven, then slice and cry tears of joy because there is no goo. None. Serves 6-8.

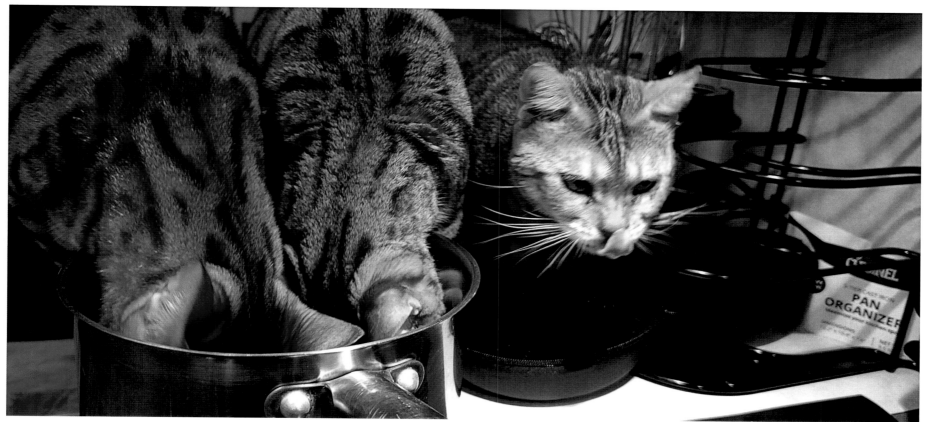

Photo Courtesy of Christopher Robinson

Miso Poached Salmon

Two things: we're all constantly hearing that we need to eat more fish. Also, cartoons taught us that cats love fish. Not mine. My cats love cake. And I really fight making fish because I'd rather make cake. Fish can be pretty challenging for a home cook in all sorts of ways, but this one might win you over. Miso is a paste of fermented soybeans with some salt and a few other things. It's loaded with all sorts of healthy minerals and vitamins and it can be your secret flavor weapon. You can find it in tubs or jars at Asian markets and some grocery stores. Poaching the salmon is a more forgiving way to cook it than grilling or baking because a) it's easy and b) it's easier to avoid overcooking and drying out the fish. A poaching liquid, like a marinade, is meant to be strongly flavored. This one is, and it may seem a bit too salty when you taste it, but it all ends happily. My daughter loves this so much that she adds extra water or broth to any leftover liquid and eats it like s soup. Which, speaking of, is a great way to use that tub of miso. Add some to your chicken or veggie soup, use to create a rub for roasting chicken, or make a salad dressing. Or, just put a dollop in a mug of boiling water and drink it.

1 ½ -2 lb. salmon fillet (if Alaskan wild-caught is an option, it's light years more delicious than farmed salmon, and it freezes well if you happen on a sale and can load up)

⅓ cup miso paste
2 cups vegetable broth*
½ onion, sliced thickly
½ lemon, sliced thinly
OPTIONAL: 2 cloves chopped garlic

In a large, deep skillet, gently whisk miso paste and broth till combined. Add onion (and garlic if using) and bring to a boil. Reduce heat to medium-low, add lemon slices. Allow to simmer for 5 minutes. Cut salmon into 4 equal-size pieces and place in pan, skin side down. Cover and cook for 5-10 minutes. Cook time depends on the thickness of the fillet. You can test for doneness by pressing your finger down on the top of the thickest part of the center of the fillet. If it flakes, it's finished. Wild-caught salmon is less fatty than farmed, so it will be ready a bit faster.

Serve the salmon over a bed of mashed potatoes, or rice, or sauteed spinach. I mean, it's even great with potato chips. Serves 4.

*2 cups vegetable broth? Who just happens to have that lying around? There's a product called *Better Than Bouillon* that's worth trying. It's a concentrated base that turns into broth when you add it to boiling water. Having a jar in the fridge makes life easier. They are not paying me to say this. I'm just all about delicious food with minimal drama and this helps you get there. A jar keeps a long time, but you'll find yourself reaching for it more often than you'd guess.

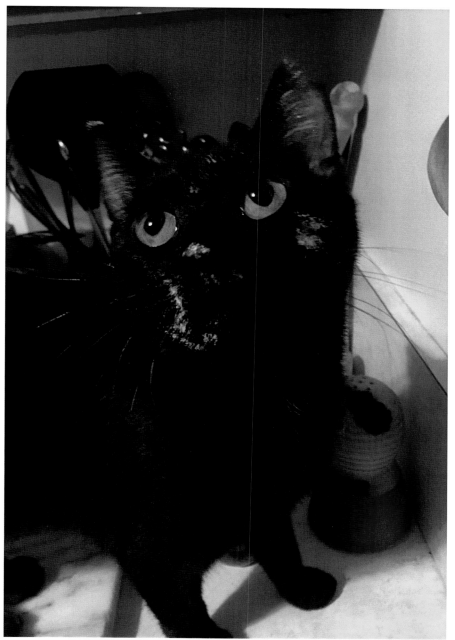

Photo Courtesy of Penny Saskia Kramer

Slow Cooker BBQ Meatloaf

I thought I hated meatloaf. There was the texture – either dry and grainy like an overcooked burger, or weirdly mushy. Then there was the ketchup-y glaze…I can't do ketchup on anything but a French fry. Then I remembered that there's no law stating that ketchup has to be involved and that a meatloaf could maybe borrow some tricks from a meatball and be more than a giant rectangular hamburger. For this recipe, I used only dried spices because, texture, and also, I have a very dramatic kid who can detect a molecule of diced onion from a mile away. Using the slow cooker not only makes it easy, it makes it less likely that you'll wind up with a brick of dried-out, overcooked meat. Plus, you can prep everything the night before and just refrigerate the uncooked loaf. Drop it in the slow cooker the next day, and 6 hours later, you've got the ultimate comfort food. For this recipe, I've suggested using your preferred store-bought bbq sauce. You can make your own, of course. It's pretty simple. It's just – sometimes it's fun to go all out in the kitchen, and sometimes it's cold and you're tired and you just want dinner. This is for that day.

2 lbs. ground beef (85% lean seems to work best for me)
2 large eggs, lightly beaten
½ cup panko breadcrumbs
½ cup milk or broth (I use unsweetened almond milk because that's what's in my fridge)
1 ½ tbsp onion powder (OR, if you live with sane people, 1 large onion, finely chopped)
1 tbsp garlic powder
1 tsp smoked paprika

1 tbsp Worcestershire sauce
1 tbsp Dijon mustard
1 tsp kosher salt
1 tsp freshly ground black pepper

For the glaze:
½ cup bbq sauce
1 tsp brown sugar
1 tsp hot sauce

Whisk together ingredients for glaze and set aside.

Pour the panko into the milk or broth and set aside.

In a large bowl, place beef, seasonings, eggs, and the milk-soaked panko breadcrumbs. Take off your rings, wash your hands, because your hands are the best kitchen tool ever invented. Gently combine all of the ingredients, being careful not to overwork the meat. Gently pat it into a loaf.

Either spray the inside of your slow cooker pan with nonstick cooking spray, wipe it with a bit of vegetable oil, or, make a little aluminum foil sling to cradle the meat. These steps make it easier to remove the finished meatloaf intact and, help with cleanup. Place the loaf into your slow cooker and spoon about half of the prepared glaze over the top. Cook on High for 4 hours, or on Low for 6 hours. Test for doneness with your instant read thermometer: an internal temp of 160° is fully cooked. Spoon or brush on remaining bbq glaze, slice. Serves 4-6. Toss any leftover slices onto the grill the next day for a seriously killer sandwich.

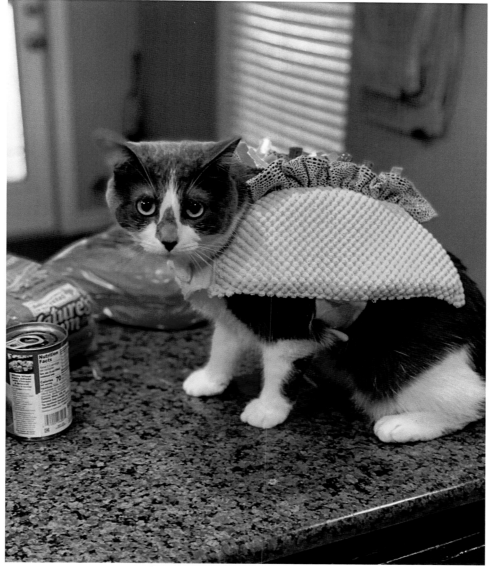

Photo Courtesy of Andrea Utenis

Broccoli & Pasta

This may be the Swiss Army knife of broccoli recipes. Made as is, it's a meatless entrée or side. Toss in some leftover roasted chicken and it's a completely different meal. Skip the pasta and serve the broccoli just as a vegetable. Chop any leftovers and add to a burrito or omelet. Orecchiette is a fun pasta for this – the word translates to 'little ear', which they kind of resemble. You can also use penne or a thin spaghetti or small shells. I've also made this with ghost broccoli aka cauliflower, and even with a mix of the two. (I called that one Haunted Broccoli in a desperate attempt to get my youngest excited about it. She just rolled her eyes. One of the cats liked it, though.)

1 head broccoli (or cauliflower), cut into florets
3 cloves garlic, thinly sliced
¼ cup extra virgin olive oil
1 tsp kosher salt
Pinch dried red pepper flakes
½ lemon

Freshly ground black pepper to taste
Freshly grated Pecorino Romano for serving

½ lb. pasta cooked according to package directions
 – reserve ½ cup of pasta cooking liquid

Bring a large pot of water to boil; add kosher salt and the broccoli/cauliflower. Cook until just barely tender, approximately 3 minutes. Drain and immediately hit it with cold running water.

Over medium-high heat, pour olive oil into a wide, deep skillet. Add garlic, red pepper flakes, and broccoli/cauliflower. Cook, stirring frequently, for 6-8 minute, or just until the vegetables begin browning at the edge. Add the ½ cup of reserved pasta water and simmer for 3-4 minutes. Taste, and season with a sprinkle of salt if needed. Add cooked pasta, combine thoroughly, and remove from heat. Sprinkle with black pepper and squeeze fresh lemon juice over entire pan. Serve hot and pass the grated cheese.

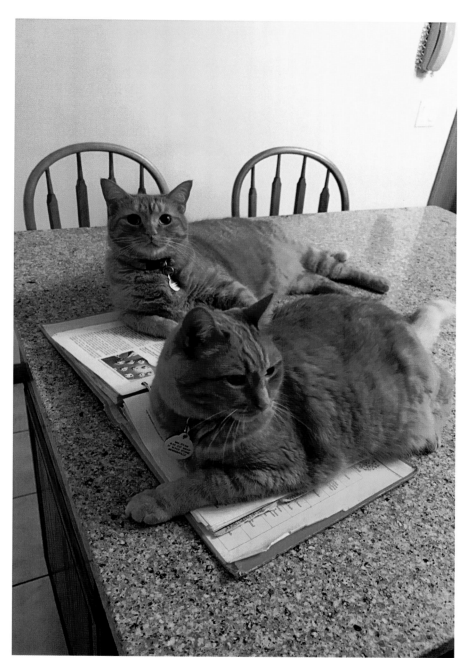

Photo Courtesy of Nancy Ryan

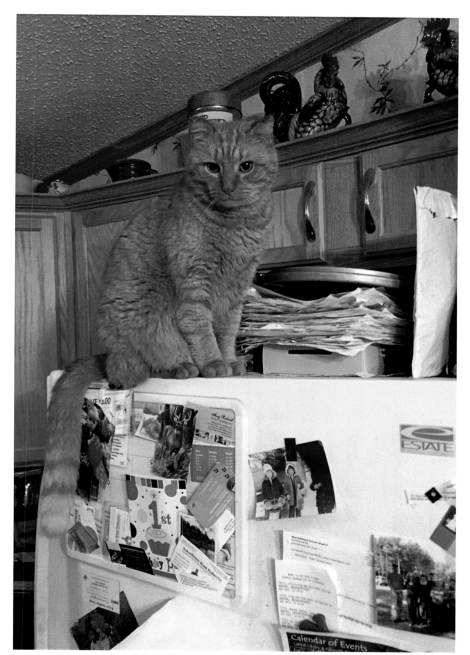

Photo Courtesy of Eileen Krom

45

Ratatouille

I grew up eating this without ever knowing its real name – my family called it "peppers and tomatoes". Wildly imaginative, right? Ratatouille is actually just a Mediterranean vegetable stew with a fancy name, and it's the best thing ever. It tastes like a summer garden. By itself, it's a vegetarian dream. It makes a killer side with grilled or roasted meat or fish. It's wonderful with polenta, rice, quinoa, couscous, or pasta. One of my favorite ways to eat it is for breakfast, topped with a couple of poached or sunny-side eggs and a mighty slab of toasted sourdough or French bread. Another name for that particular preparation is 'shakshuka'. Something I love about this dish – and really, cooking in general – is the way recipes migrate across geography and cultures, changing and evolving along the way. This spicy vegetable stew originated in northern Africa and made its way to southern Europe, Israel, the Middle East…and your kitchen. How cool is that? I had to create a written recipe for my family's version of this, but after you make it once, you sure won't ever need me again. You might like your veggies diced into smaller pieces, or maybe you hate eggplant so much that we can't even talk about it. That's fine. This is about to be your recipe, made your way.

5 tbsp olive oil
1 medium onion, chopped
5 cloves garlic, finely chopped
2 bell peppers, seeded and sliced into 1 inch pieces
1 medium eggplant, washed, unpeeled, quartered, and cut into 1-inch pieces
2 medium or 1 large zucchini, washed, unpeeled, halved lengthwise, cut into 1-inch pieces
1 medium yellow squash, washed, unpeeled, halved lengthwise, cut into 1-inch pieces

1 28 oz can whole San Marzano tomatoes
3 ½ cups water
½ cup dry red wine
1 tbsp kosher salt
1 tsp dried basil OR 1 tbsp fresh basil leaves, torn into small pieces
1 tsp dried rosemary OR 1 tbsp fresh rosemary leaves, finely chopped
½ tsp dried thyme OR ½ tbsp fresh thyme leaves
1 dried bay leaf
OPTIONAL: ¼ tsp dried red pepper flakes

In a large, deep pan or skillet, add 2 tbsp of olive oil and sauté onion and garlic over medium heat until just translucent – about 5 minutes. Add bell pepper and sauté, stirring often, for 10 minutes. If needed, add another 2-3 tbsp olive oil along with half of the eggplant, zucchini, and squash and continue to cook, stirring frequently. All of these vegetables contain a lot of water and as that liquid releases, you'll have more room in the pan to add the remaining vegetables. Do that, stirring often for another few minutes. Now, using your hands, crush and break up the tomatoes and add those, along with the water and wine, to the pan. Stir in basil, rosemary, thyme, pepper flakes, bay leaf, and salt. Bring to a boil, stir, and reduce heat to low. Simmer gently for at least 30 minutes. Taste and add salt if needed. Serve with a swirl of good quality extra-virgin olive oil. Serves 4 as a main, 6-8 as a side, and freezes like a dream. NOTE: this is even better the next day; refrigerate the finished stew, and warm it up before serving.

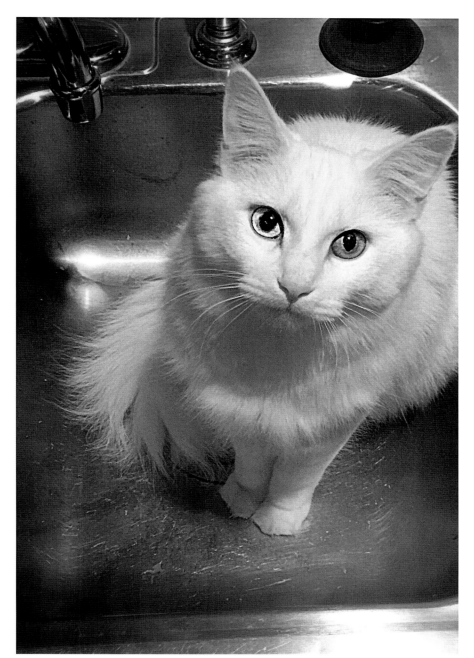

Photo Courtesy of Misty Tracy

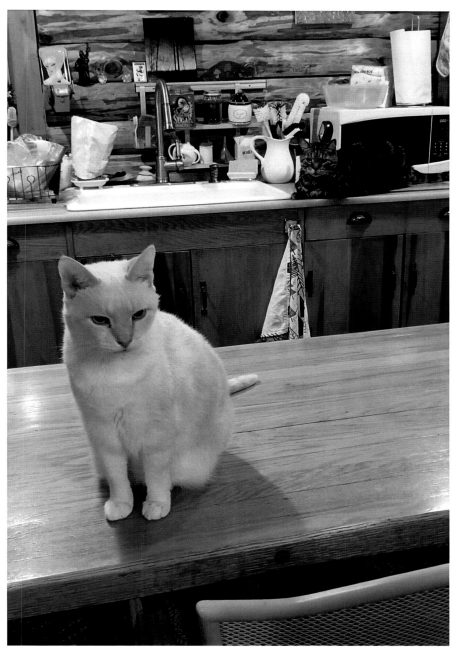

Photo Courtesy of Deborah Seidner

Arroz con Pollo a la Anubis

Tony Garcia is half Italian, half Puerto Rican and (mostly) cool with sharing his kitchen with a huge, codependent scavenger of a cat. He's also a really good cook, which isn't surprising given that his father, born and raised in Puerto Rico, was a chef. Tony's mother and grandmother were the kind of tiny, devoted little Italian kitchen wizards that really thrive in the rich soil of Long Island. He was their prince, fussed over and doted upon and fed and fed and fed to the point where you'd be right to wonder how such a royal personage ever learned to boil water, much less to cook. Well, genetics are a powerful thing and so is Tony's wife, Donna. He traded his princely life for a wedding ring and got himself into the kitchen. This recipe is one he's adapted for the Instant Pot or pressure cooker of your choice. Tony's family likes a lot of rice relative to the amount of chicken called for, but the recipe is super flexible, and you can adjust the ratios according to your preferences. As for the codependent cat, Anubis, he lives to steal food off of the counters and is in cahoots with the dog, Rain. Anubis snatches the snack and he and Rain sneak off to feast together. It's a beautiful friendship.

2 tbsp extra virgin olive oil

1 medium yellow onion, diced (about 1 cup)

1 medium green bell pepper, diced (about 1 cup)

4 cups rice (rinsed and drained)

1 packet Goya Sazon Con Azrafan

Goya Adobo

1 32 oz container low-sodium chicken broth

2 lbs. boneless, skinless chicken breasts

Cut chicken into bite-size chunks; season liberally on both sides with the Goya Adobo.

Set Instant Pot to sauté setting. When it comes to temperature, add onions and pepper. Sauté for 3-5b minutes, until pepper is softened, and onion is translucent.

Add chicken and sauté 5-8 minutes or until the meat is no longer pink.

Stir in rice and mix well with chicken and vegetables. Add broth to pot and stir in the packet of Sazon Con Azafran.

Seal lid of pot and set to Rice setting. When cooking is complete, allow for a natural release of steam for 5-7 minutes, then carefully vent the remaining steam using the quick release method. (Always be careful when releasing steam from your pressure cooker. Use a utensil to push the valve into the Release position. You can also place a kitchen towel over the vent and safely capture the steam that way.)

Serve in small bowls. Yields about 8 1 ½ cup servings.

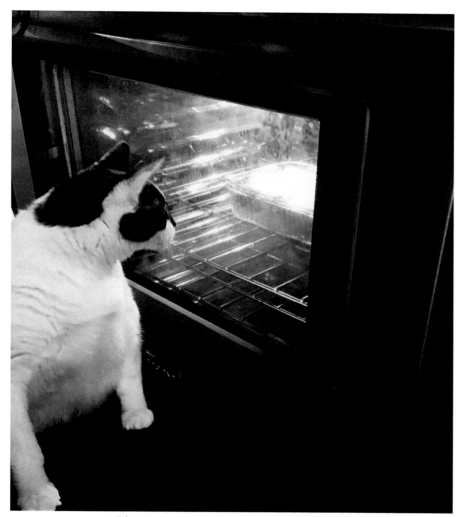

Photo Courtesy of Melissa Chenault

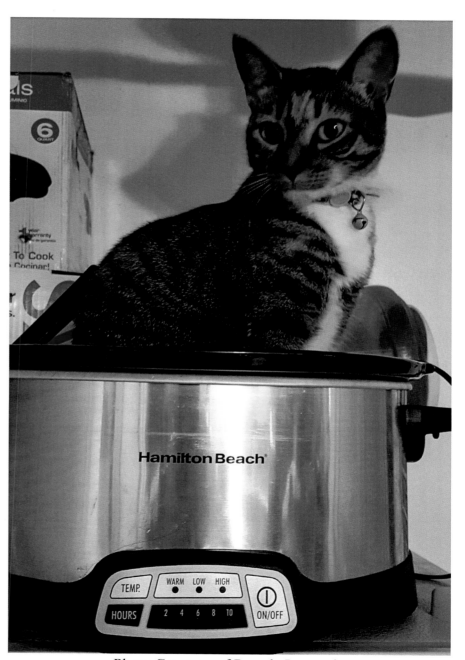

Photo Courtesy of Pamela Langevin

Sausage & Veggie Roast

Some days you walk into the kitchen and just don't feel like making any effort. AT ALL. Everyone's whiny or grumbling or hissing and yowling, nothing easy looks good and nothing good looks easy. This recipe has your back. It basically rounds up a whole bunch of random and orphaned vegetables and that stray package of sausage in the back of the freezer and turns them into a one-pan savory meal. It's all helped along by a seriously brawny vinaigrette that can also double as a salad dressing for sturdy greens, fresh spinach, and sliced, boiled potatoes. You can substitute vegetables based on what you have on hand. You can whip this up right now and pop it in the oven, or you can prep it ahead and let it all marinate in the fridge for 2-24 hours. Not to be bossy, but I think you'll want a big glass of red and a loaf of some sort of rustic bread to mop up the juices. Scramble up some eggs with the leftovers for breakfast the next day.

Vinaigrette:

1 cup extra virgin olive oil
¼ cup balsamic vinegar
¼ cup whole grain mustard*
2 tsp honey

½ tsp salt
½ tsp black pepper
¼ tsp crushed red pepper
2 cloves garlic, finely minced

1 cup cherry or grape tomatoes
1 cup carrots, peeled, bite-size chunks
1 cup parsnip, peeled, bite-size chunks
1 bell pepper, cored, seeded, bite-sized chunks
½ - 1 head ghost broccoli aka cauliflower
   OR broccoli, cut into florets

2 cups red cabbage, coarsely shredded
1 lb. red potatoes, unpeeled, cut into wedges
1 med-large sweet potato, peeled, cut into wedges
1 large onion, peeled, sliced in thick wedges
2 lb. sausage, thawed. Smoked, brats, Italian – your choice. Cut links into thirds.

Prepare the vinaigrette by combining all ingredients in a large glass jar. Seal it up and shake it like crazy to emulsify. Is this a classic technique? No, but I'm a crazy cat lady, not a French chef. Alternatively, you can put all of the ingredients except the olive oil into a bowl, and then slowly pour the olive oil in as you gently and thoroughly whisk to combine. Either way, don't worry about the dressing separating. Just shake or whisk it again. You can't hurt it.

Preheat oven to 375°. Place the sausages and all of the veggies in a large bowl. Pour the vinaigrette over and toss, making sure everything is coated. (If making ahead, seal tightly and refrigerate until ready to roast.)

Line a large baking sheet with aluminum foil – easier clean up. Spread the sausage and vegetables in a single layer. Roast for 20 minutes, then give it all a big stir with a slotted spoon, making sure to keep it all in a single layer. Roast 20-25 minutes longer, until everything is browned and caramelized. Pile onto a platter and serve with loads of crusty bread. Serves 4-6.

*Dijon mustard can be substituted. The whole grain just has a bit more oomph.

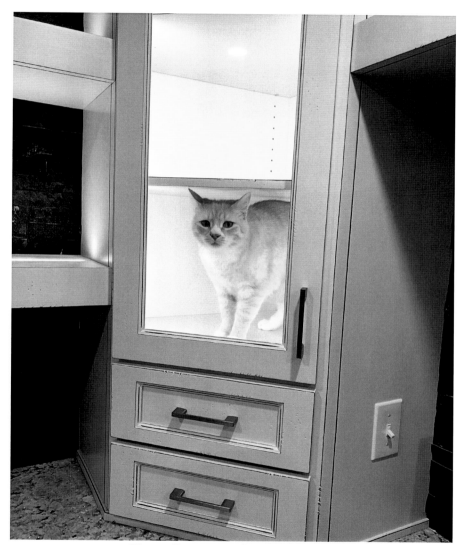

Photo Courtesy of Kristin Reed

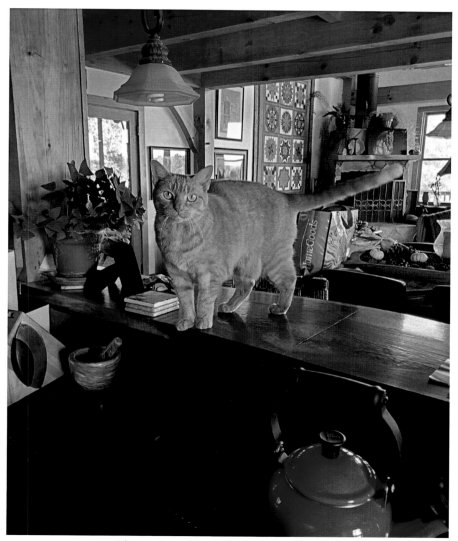

Photo Courtesy of Barbara Shifflett

Kerri's Friendship Soup

Kerri Green is a about a million different things and she's great at all of them: mom, wife, friend, cat lady, writer. She's far too humble to say this herself, so you'll have to trust me. Her home is northern California is like the Tardis in Dr. Who: it may look small on the outside, but her front door opens into a near-infinite space of love and welcome and coziness. Also, some chaos at times, because all of the homiest places always have a big dash of that. Her friend Amanda brought this soup after Kerri had been in a car accident. Amanda just knew, somehow, what was needed. Kerri says, "She brought me more than simple soup that day. She brought warmth, and her big, beautiful smile…that soup drop-off began what would grow into one of the most meaningful friendships of my life. Over the years I've made changes to this Friendship Soup. Her offering, her gift of love, and some things of my own that I've added – this soup is a true picture of friendship. Every time I make it, I remember a friend that showed up and helped to heal me. Now I'm sharing it with you." Your heart needs this soup and your home will smell amazing while it cooks. Before I forget, I must also tell you that Kerri's cat, Seuess, is a majestic cloud of charcoal fur in search of a snuggle. You. Would. Die.

1 tbsp olive oil
1 yellow onion, chopped
4 cloves garlic, minced
1 lb. carrots, peeled, sliced into coins
6 stalks celery, sliced
6 cups (approximately) chicken broth
2 ½- 3lbs baby golden potatoes, unpeeled, bite-size pieces

1 large rotisserie chicken, cut into cubes
2-3 tbsp fresh sage, chopped
1 tbsp fresh rosemary
3 sprigs fresh thyme
Juice of 1-2 fresh lemons
Salt & pepper to taste

Place oil and onions into a large stock pot and cook over medium heat until the onions soften and start to become translucent – 3-5 minutes. Add in garlic and cook 1 minute more.

Add carrots, celery, potatoes, cubed chicken, broth, and herbs. Increase heat, boiling until potatoes are soft, approximately 20-25 minutes.

Remove thyme sprigs and add lemon juice. (Kerri suggests starting with one lemon and adjusting to your taste. She also notes that lemon can be omitted completely, but it really does add something special to the finished soup.)

Season with salt and pepper and serve!

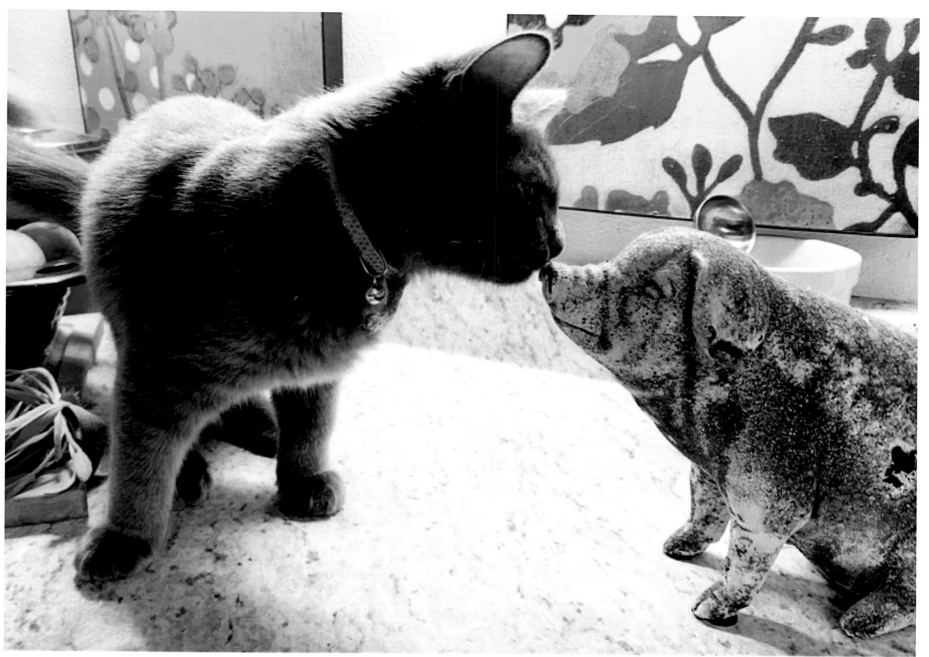

Photo Courtesy of Kerri Green

Il Tacchino di Mario alla Bolognese

A fancy name because Mario is a fancy cat. A cat who loves riding in the car so much that he cries at the door until his humans relent and go get the keys. Mario's humans, Cyndi and Scott Conrow, along with their son, Nate, weren't even sure they wanted a cat. They definitely didn't want a cat who jumped onto the kitchen counters. And Scott was allergic. It took a Devon Rex to steal their hearts, and where there is one, there's almost always another. Enter Princess Peach. Now they have to take defensive measures any time they want to grate a block of cheese. But what a small price to pay for a cat who loves the road? And would Scott really want to live even one more day without his special cat backpack? Cyndi used to be active in a rescue program for the Devon Rex breed, but at the moment she's got her hands full with a teenage son and a cat who just wants to take to the open road. Lucky for us, she found time to make this quick and delicious pasta.

1 lb. spaghetti, uncooked
2 tbsp olive oil
1 lb. ground turkey*
1 large onion, chopped
4 cloves garlic, minced
1 tbsp dried oregano
¼ tsp red pepper flakes
2 tbsp tomato paste
1 cup hearty red wine (Chianti, Pinot Noir, or Merlot)

1 28 oz can crushed tomatoes
2 tbsp fresh basil, chopped OR 2 tsp dried basil
   PLUS 2 tbsp fresh basil, chopped, for garnish
½ tsp salt =/- to taste
½ tsp pepper - +/- to taste
½ cup heavy cream OPTIONAL
½ cup grated Asiago cheese (can substitute Parmesan)

Cook the spaghetti according to package instructions.

In a large skillet or pan over medium-high heat, heat olive oil. Add the turkey, and cook thoroughly, using a wooden spoon or utensil to break the meat up as it cooks. Add onion and garlic to the meat, cooking just until the onion becomes translucent.

Add the oregano, red pepper flakes, and tomato paste. (If you've never tried concentrated tomato paste in a tube, now is the time. It adds a lot of flavor.) Stir in the red wine and cook until most of the liquid has cooked off – about 5 minutes. Add crushed tomatoes, basil, salt and pepper and stir. Bring to a boil, then reduce heat to medium-low. Cover and simmer for 20 minutes. IF using heavy cream, stir it in. Taste, and adjust salt and pepper if needed.

Add cooked pasta to the sauce and toss well. Top with grated cheese and fresh basil. Serves 6.

*if you prefer, ground beef or a plant-based meat substitute can be used instead of turkey

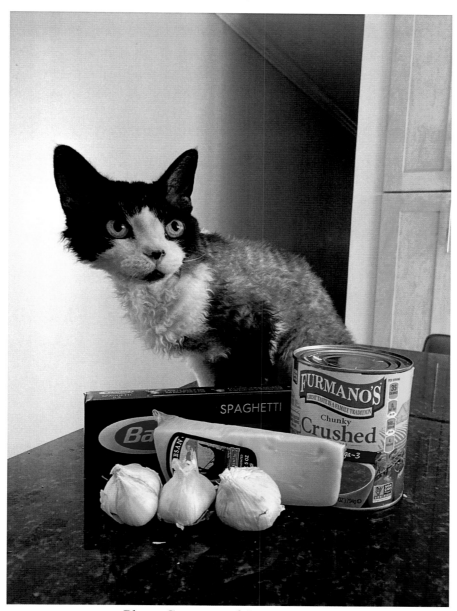

Photo Courtesy of Scott Conrow

Vidalia Onion Savory Tart

I love pie and pizza in any form, and a quick rustic fruit tart is my go-to move for an easy homemade dessert. So why not pay tribute to all of those things? You can use any onions for this dish, of course, but if you've never cooked with a sweet onion like the Vidalia, that marvel of South Georgia, give it a try. The bacon lends plenty of smoky flavor, and the prosciutto adds a salty kick. Just pre-bake your homemade or store-bought crust before filling so that the bottom isn't soggy. This makes for a very fancy breakfast or brunch but add a green salad and you've got dinner. If you use a tart pan with a removable bottom, the end result will be so pretty that you'll almost hate to cut into it. Almost. You can also make this in a standard pie plate or glass baking dish. You can even freestyle and do a rustic version on a parchment paper-lined baking sheet. As for the cheese, I'm super committed to Gruyere, but never let fear of a substitution keep you from cooking. Use what you have – cheddar, mozzarella, Jack, Swiss – you can't hurt it. (For a meatless option, omit the pork and increase butter to 4 tbsp).

1 ½ lbs. Vidalia or other onion, peeled, sliced thinly

2 tbsp butter (4, if omitting bacon)

6 strips thick-cut bacon or 8 strips regular bacon, diced

4 oz prosciutto, sliced into ribbons

1 cup gruyere cheese, grated OR 1 cup of grated cheese

¾ cup light cream or half-and-half

1 large egg

3 egg yolks

½ tsp freshly ground black pepper, plus more to taste

½ tsp salt

½ tsp ground nutmeg OR ground thyme (Ina Garten's mac and cheese recipe taught me the power of pairing nutmeg with Gruyere. Give it a shot.)

1 sheet of purchased pie dough OR homemade if you're up for it

Over medium heat, cook the bacon till crisp. Remove from pan and set aside. Add 2 tbsp butter to the bacon drippings, along with all of the sliced onion. Reduce heat to medium-low and cook the onions until they are soft, translucent, and caramelized. This will take approximately forever, or 45 minutes to an hour. Stir the onions periodically and do not let them burn. Remove the onions from the pan (you can even do this step a day or so ahead and just refrigerate until ready to assemble the tart.)

Preheat oven to 350°. Line your pan with pie crust. Top with aluminum foil and pie weights or dried beans. Bake for 25 minutes. Remove the foil and weights and allow to cool.

Reduce oven temperature to 325°. In a medium bowl, whisk together cream, egg, and egg yolks with salt, pepper, and nutmeg or thyme. Gently fold the bacon and prosciutto into the caramelized onions. Spread this mixture evenly over the prebaked crust. Sprinkle the grated cheese over the onion and pork layer. Carefully drizzle the egg and cream over the entire tart. Bake for 50 minutes to 1 hour. (Slide a baking sheet onto the bottom rack of your oven to catch any drips and to make cleanup easier.) Cool for 10 minutes before removing from tart pan (if using – and if needed, use the tip of a sharp knife to separate the pastry from the fluted side of the pan.) Serve warm. Serves 6 as a meal.

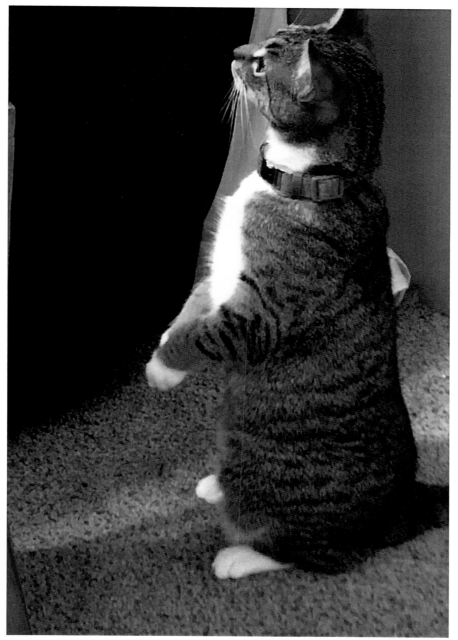

Photo Courtesy of Joann Goins

Is THIS the Gumbo?

My late mother-in-law was born in Mississippi. When she was very small, a tornado slammed into town and swallowed up her daddy. She went on to be raised by a loving stepfather in Covington, Louisiana, studied nursing at Vanderbilt, traveled the world with her husband, and left this life remembered by all as a woman possessed of both grace and a fearsome inner strength. She could control chaos with the lifting of a single eyebrow and could put even the most hyper kid to sleep in minutes with her legendary monotone reading of Brighty of the Grand Canyon. I inherited her little dog and my husband's memories of her gumbo. Which I've been trying to recreate ever since. But let's get back to that tornado. If that had happened in my family, it's the only thing any of us would talk about for the next hundred years. But my husband's family? "Oh honey, that was such a long time ago." Really? REALLY? Oh, okay. And no one wrote down that gumbo recipe either? Got it. This is not Nana Sarah's gumbo, but it's the closest I've gotten. The last time I cooked for her my cats were all up in the business and as you might expect from a woman with her life experiences, she didn't care a bit. Or if she did, she was far too polite and gracious to say so. What a true queen.

1 large onion, diced

1 green bell pepper, diced

1 bunch celery, including the leaves, finely chopped

1 cup fresh parsley, finely chopped

4 green onions, thinly sliced

3 cloves garlic peeled and smashed (use the flat of knife blade and whomp it. So satisfying.)

3 tbsp vegetable oil

1 lb. andouille sausage, sliced into ¼ inch thick coins

4 cups cooked chicken (rotisserie, poached, leftover from roasting – your call)

2 cups peeled, cooked shrimp

8-10 cups chicken broth

2 tbsp Cajun seasoning*

File powder

Optional: 4 cups cooked white rice

For the roux:

1 cup all-purpose flour

1 cup vegetable oil

The trick here, as I learned the hard way, is the roux. It's not difficult, but it calls for the kind of patience and constant stirring you'd expect from risotto. Place flour and oil into a large, heavy stockpot. Over medium-low heat (and watch it, because a burnt roux is awful and fit only for the trash), cook, stirring continuously until you're completely over it and ready to quit, about 45 minutes. At least. The roux at this point will be a deep, rich brown, very thick and syrupy. Set aside.

In a cast iron skillet over medium, sauté the andouille coins until lightly browned on both sides. Set aside. Add 2-3 tbsp vegetable oil to the pan, and sauté the onion, celery, and bell pepper aka the holy trinity of Cajun cooking, until softened. Add the smashed garlic to the pan, stir, remove from heat. Set aside.

Add the chicken broth to the prepared roux in the stockpot, pouring slowly and whisking gently to minimize lumpiness. Add sausage, cooked chicken, and the sauteed vegetables. Stir in Cajun seasoning. Simmer on low for at least 30 minutes, stirring occasionally. I generally let it simmer for 45-60 minutes. 5 minutes before serving, add 2 tbsp file powder, cooked shrimp, parsley and sliced green onions. Stir. (Another thing I learned the hard way: adding the file too soon makes the texture of the gumbo stringy and weird.)

Serve over cooked rice, if you like. Folks who love spicy foods can add hot sauce or a bit more file at the table. Serves 4-6.

*Cajun seasoning is sold at grocery stores, but you can easily make your own if you can't find it. There are recipes online and it's all pretty basic spices you probably have on hand and need to use up anyway: paprika, garlic and onion powder, thyme, oregano, cayenne, salt and pepper.

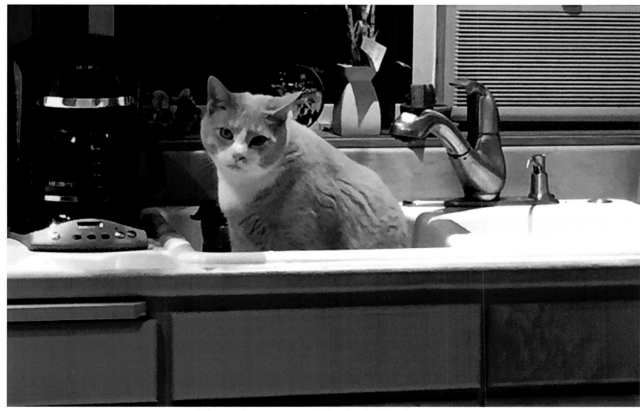

Photo Courtesy of Kimberly Waltemate

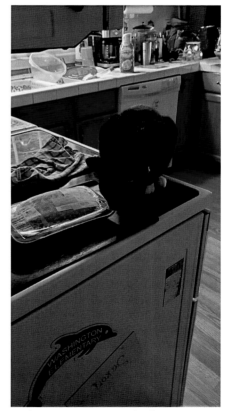

Photo Courtesy of Lisa Saxon

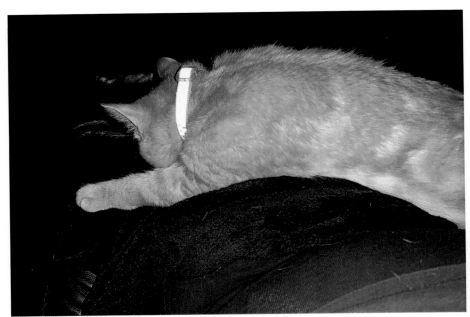

Photo Courtesy of Meredith Chandler

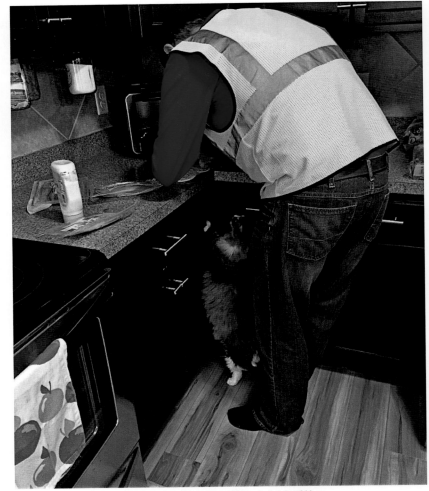

Photo Courtesy of Knicki Miller

Sweets

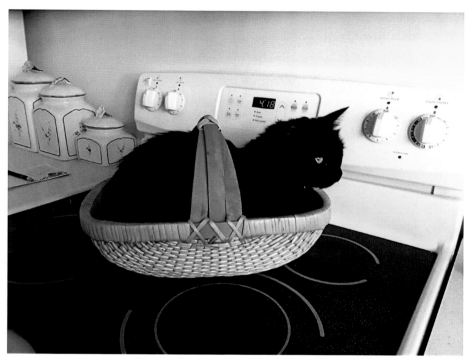

Photo Courtesy of Barbara Biro

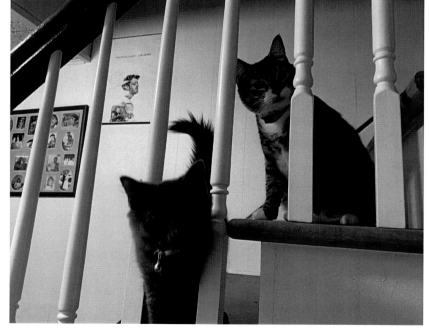

Photo Courtesy of Bonnie Bee

Grandmom Blackhair's Apple Cake

This recipe is super forgiving, and easy, even if you've never baked from scratch. It's fancy enough for a holiday dessert, but not so sweet that you can't eat it for breakfast. My grandmom baked this any time she had a handful of past-their-prime apples rolling around in the fridge. I do the same, but my favorites for this cake are tart Granny Smiths. If your cats are groveling carb fiends like mine, hide this cake while it cools, or the little monsters will gnaw the top right off of it.

4 large eggs (room temp)
2 cups white sugar, plus 2 tbsp set aside
1 cup vegetable oil
3 tsp baking powder
3 cups all-purpose flour, plus 1 tbsp set aside
¼ tsp salt
2 tsp pure vanilla extract
½ cup orange juice (or pineapple juice)

4 cups apple, peeled, cored, thinly sliced
   – think potato chips – (approx. 4 large apples)
1 tbsp cinnamon
¼ tsp ground nutmeg

Topping:
2 tbsp confectioner sugar
¼ tsp cinnamon

Preheat oven to 350°. Grease and flour a 10-inch tube cake pan. (You can also use an angel food pan, or a Bundt pan – just make sure it's large enough. Aim for 16 cup capacity.)

Toss apple slices with 1 tbsp cinnamon and 1/4 tsp nutmeg. Set aside.

Mix flour, baking powder, and salt together in medium-sized bowl. In a separate bowl, using a hand or stand mixer, beat eggs, sugar, and oil together until smooth and well combined. Fold in dry ingredients, alternating with juice and vanilla extract, until just combined and smooth.

You're going to layer the batter and apples – 3 layers of batter, 2 of apples. Pour first layer of batter into prepared pan. Using your hands, carefully place a layer of sliced apples on top, sprinkling a bit of the reserved flour over the fruit. Repeat process with a second layer of batter, and a second layer of fruit. Top with a final layer of batter.

Bake for one hour. I use a piece of dry spaghetti to check for doneness – any liquid batter on the pasta means you need about another 5 minutes bake time. A bit of moist crumb is okay and means you're ready to haul it out of the oven. Cool 10 minutes in pan, then invert onto a wire rack and let cool for at least 45 minutes. Sift or sieve confectioner sugar and cinnamon mixture over entire cake before serving.

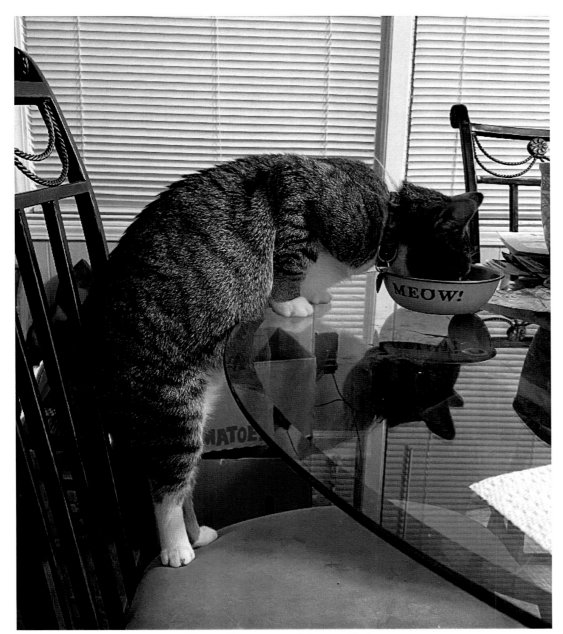

Photo Courtesy of Joann Goins

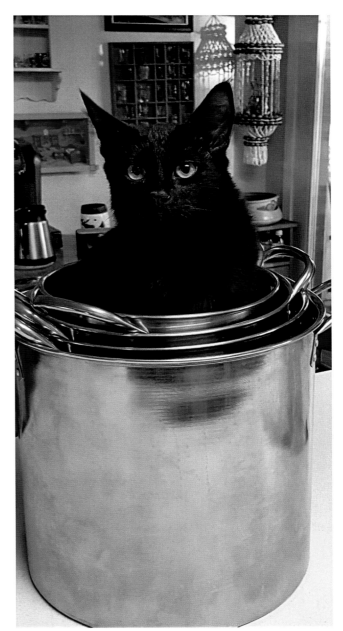

Photo Courtesy of Cheri Thomas

The Stolen Cheesecake

My gram had a real frenemy relationship with the glam divorcee who lived across the street. This was back when glam divorcees were far scarcer than today, and this particular neighbor was a bit of a show-off, according to family lore. She had painted concrete statues on her front lawn – a jaunty burro AND the Virgin Mary – and an apparently amazing cheesecake recipe which she hoarded like a goblin. So, one summer night when she was out of town, my gram and my aunt sneaked over, filched the key from under the backdoor mat, let themselves in, and rummaged through her kitchen till they found her recipe. From that day forward, The Stolen Cheesecake became a family dessert tradition. About a million years later, I grew up and figured out that the original recipe must surely have been printed on a package of Kraft's Philadelphia-brand cream cheese, adapted and tweaked over time by these crazy gangsta ladies. Whatever. It's easy and delicious, and maybe even worth breaking and entering.

3 8 oz packages cream cheese, softened
    (Philadelphia brand, if you want to be legit)
3 eggs
1 ½ tsp pure vanilla extract, divided
1 tsp orange zest*
1 tbsp fresh orange juice*

1 scant cup white sugar plus 3 tbsp set aside
1 ½ cup sour cream
1 cup vanilla wafer cookie crumbs OR graham cracker OR butter cookies
3 tbsp butter, melted

*lemon zest and juice can be substituted

Preheat oven to 325°.

Combine cookie crumbs with the melted butter and 3 tbsp of sugar. Press into the bottom of a 9-inch springform pan and bake for 10 minutes.

Using a hand or stand mixer on medium speed, beat cream cheese, ½ tsp vanilla extract, citrus zest and juice, and ¾ cup sugar until well combined and smooth. On low speed, add eggs, 1 at a time, until just blended. Pour over prepared crust.

Bake 1 hour, or until center is almost set. (I start checking at 50 minutes). While baking, mix sour cream, 1 tsp vanilla extract, and ¾ cup sugar until thoroughly combined. Spread sour cream mixture very carefully over top of baked cheesecake, and pop back into the oven for 10 minutes. Remove, allow to cool for another 10 minutes. Gently run the blade of a sharp knife around the rim of the pan, remove the springform, and refrigerate the cheesecake for 4-6 hours before serving.

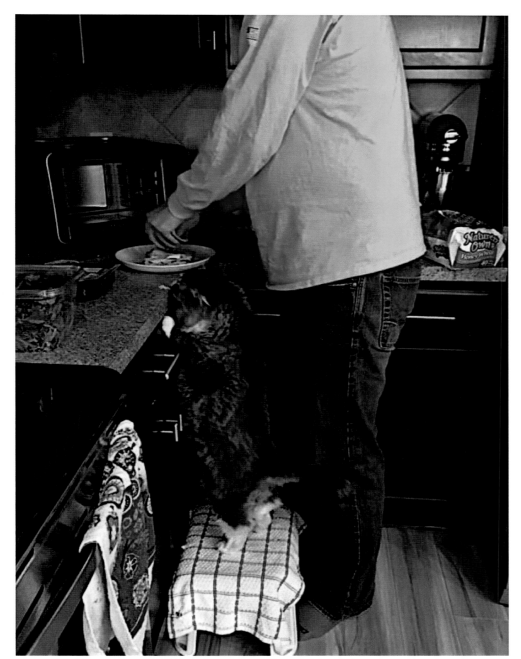

Photo Courtesy of Knicki Miller

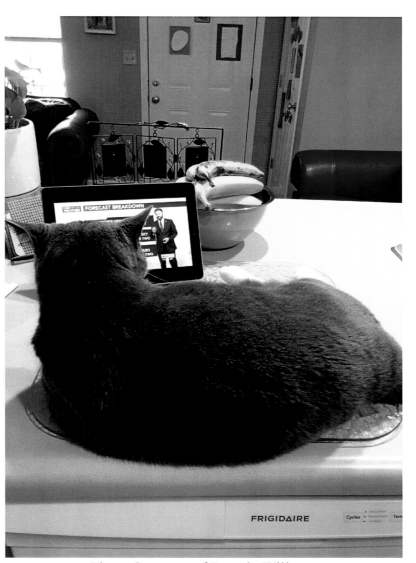

Photo Courtesy of Pamela Willeroy

Miss Jewel's Fruit Cobbler

Miss Jewel was a truly great Southern lady and a legendary home cook. Her son, my BFF Rick, learned at her side and he and I have been cooking together for years. I could fill a book with her recipes alone, and all of them would be among the most delicious things you'd ever tasted. This cobbler is amazing with any stone fruit, berries, apples – fresh, frozen, canned, or even a combination of fruits will work. Just be sure to thoroughly drain frozen or canned fruit before adding to batter. This particular version calls for fresh blackberries. Truvy, in the movie Steel Magnolias, makes a version with canned fruit cocktail and even that is probably to die for. But fresh berries? Yes, ma'am! This is painfully easy to make and so rich and yummy that you could skip the whipped cream or ice cream, but why? Why do you want to make yourself unhappy? Miss Jewel don't play like that. Have yourself some whipped cream. Oh, and trust me: no cat would dare to set a paw on her kitchen counters. How could you even suggest such a thing? Bless your heart.

1 cup self-rising flour
1 cup white sugar
1 cup whole milk
1 stick unsalted butter
1 tbsp pure vanilla extract

18-24 oz fresh blackberries*
2 tbsp brown sugar (optional)
2 tbsp honey dissolved in 1 cup hot water (optional)

Slide a 9x13 glass baking dish into the oven and preheat to 350°. Very carefully place the stick of butter into the dish and let it melt and brown. This should take about 20 minutes. Why this step? Browning the butter evaporates the water, concentrates the butter flavor, and adds a nutty, mellow depth to the cobbler. It's a huge payoff for so little effort. If you're in a wild hurry, of course you can just melt the butter and get on with it but taking that extra bit of time to let it brown could possibly change your life.

While that's working, taste the berries. If they're a little anemic or too tart, give them a soak in the warm honey syrup while your butter browns. Drain.

In a medium bowl, combine flour and sugar. Whisk in milk and vanilla extract. The batter will have the thin consistency of pancake batter. Very carefully remove the hot baking dish from the oven and pour the batter in. Do not stir! Place the fruit into the batter and again, no stirring. (The batter will rise around the fruit as it bakes.) If you like, sprinkle brown sugar over the top – there's just something magical about brown sugar with blackberries. Bake 40-60 minutes, until golden brown and set. Serve warm with whipped cream and/or ice cream.

*if using peaches, plums, or nectarines, go with at least 2 cups of peeled, sliced fruit

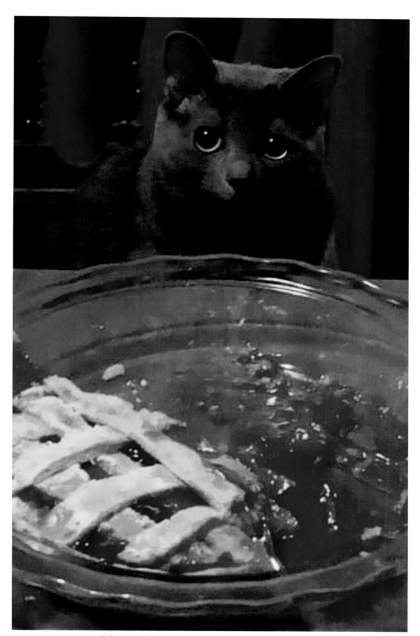

Photo Courtesy of Devin Stanfield

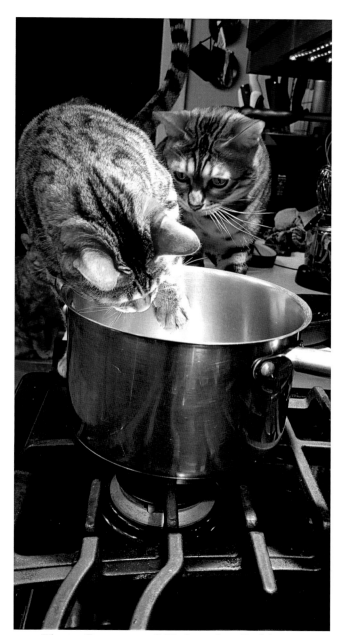

Photo Courtesy of Christopher Robinson

Grandma Jacque's Lebkuchen

Let's get one thing straight: Grandma Jacque will not tolerate cats in the kitchen. She'd rather they weren't even in the house, okay? But definitely not anywhere near her kitchen counters and God forbid, never near food she's preparing. Hard no. These cookies are a little spicy, though not as much as gingerbread. Crunchy with a bit of softness at the center, Grandma Jacque would bake them by the literal thousands and ship them out – my kids couldn't wait for the box to arrive so they could decorate them. The dough is stiff and calls for the kind of brute strength that comes naturally to Wisconsin grandmothers and possibly, I don't know, professional assassins. This recipe makes a lot of cookies. I mean, A LOT of cookies. No one knows exactly how many because that is part of the magic of Jacque's kitchen.

1 ½ cup dark molasses
¾ cup honey
1 ½ cup white sugar
1 cup unsalted butter, plus 2 tbsp
4 level tsp baking soda
1 tsp ground cloves
¾ tsp ground cardamom
4 eggs, separated. Set the yolks aside and lightly
   beat the whites to very soft peaks

1 cup finely chopped nuts (walnuts or pecans)
4-6 cups all-purpose flour (or more –
   I KNOW it sounds crazy. Just keep the whole bag out.)

Glaze:
1 cup confectioner sugar
2-3 tbsp fresh lemon juice
Pinch salt

In a large saucepan over medium-low heat, melt butter, molasses, honey, and sugar. Add cardamom, cloves, baking soda, and about a half cup of the flour. Stir. Remove from heat and fold in the yolks and the lightly beaten egg whites. Gently stir in the chopped nuts.

Now, start adding in flour. Jacque says, "as much as you can." The dough will be a bit sticky. Cover with plastic wrap and refrigerate overnight.

To bake, remove dough from refrigerator. It will be hard. Jacque cuts it into sections in the bowl and pries each section out. This may be a workout, FYI. Allow the dough to come to room temp before even attempting to wrestle with it.

Preheat the oven to 350°. Lightly flour a marble slab and marble rolling pin and dust each section of dough with flour as well. Roll dough to desired thickness – ¼ inch makes for a nice, crisp cookie. Using a 2-3-inch cookie cutter – or Jacque's go-to, a shot glass – cut the dough and place onto parchment paper-lined baking sheets. Space cookies about 1-1 ½ inches apart. Bake 7-10 minutes, depending on thickness.

Cool thoroughly on a wire rack. To make the glaze, whisk the powdered sugar, lemon juice, and salt till smooth. Spread on cooled cookies. If adding sprinkles or other decorations, add those while glaze is wet – it sets up very quickly. Both the dough and the cookies freeze well. Which is great, because you're going to have a lot. So, so many.

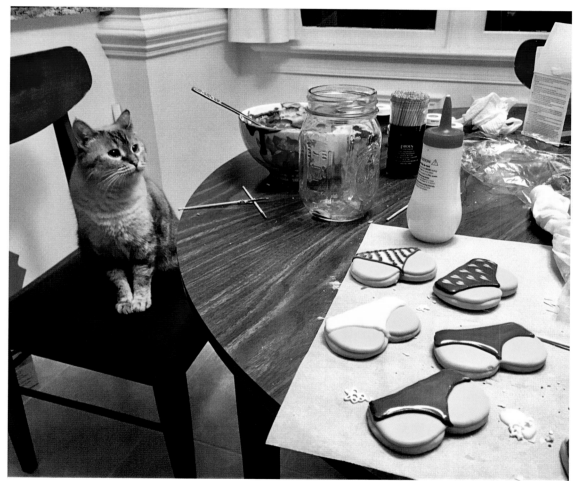

Photo Courtesy of Mary Kathrine Snow

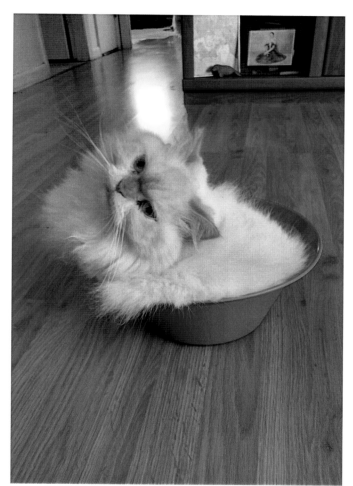

Photo Courtesy of Lucinda Sears

The Purrrrfect Chocolate Cake

Cat lady Jenn Jackson started out with no cats, and now has 3 because that's how cats work. Jenn admits, "I should not be a crazy cat lady because I'm asthmatic and ridiculously allergic to cats, but I gave up on that a long time ago. I mean, their sweet faces! I LOVE my cats. So, I ignore the scowls from my doctors when I tell them I have 3, and just continue my regimen of allergy meds. My cats and our rituals keep me sane when the humans around me are driving me nuts." Jenn is an amazing baker – she used to co-own a restaurant and made most of the desserts herself. Now she bakes for fun, and you know you're living right when she rolls up with a special cake for your birthday. This recipe really is the perfect indulgence, whether you're celebrating something special or just celebrating the fact that you have a face to stuff it into.

For cake layers:

½ cup fine quality semisweet chocolate chips
   (Jenn recommends Ghirardelli,
   because only the best will do for crazy cat people)
1 ½ cups strong-brewed hot coffee
3 cups granulated white sugar
2 ½ cups all-purpose flour
1 ½ cups unsweetened cocoa powder
   (you can't go wrong with Ghirardelli or Hershey's Dark)

2 tsp baking soda
¾ tsp baking powder
1 ¼ tsp salt
3 large eggs
¾ cup vegetable oil
1 ½ cups buttermilk, shake well
¾ tsp pure vanilla extract

For ganache frosting:

2 cups fine quality semisweet chocolate chips
   (Jenn reminds you that you are a Cat Queen/King
   and you deserve only the best: Ghirardelli.)
1 cup heavy cream

2 tbsp granulated white sugar
2 tbsp light corn syrup
½ stick butter, cut into 1 inch pieces
OPTIONAL: ½ cup mini chocolate chips for garnish

Preheat oven to 300°. Spray two 9x2 round cake pans with nonstick cooking spray. Line the bottom of each with a round of parchment paper, then spray the paper.

Pour hot coffee into a large measuring cup and add ½ cup chocolate chips. Stir until chocolate is melted and smooth. Set aside.

In a large bowl, combine, sugar, flour, cocoa, baking soda, baking powder, and salt. With a large whisk gently mix dry ingredients by hand until well blended.

If you have a standing mixer, now's the time to use it! If not, a hand mixer is fine. In a separate large bowl, beat eggs on medium speed until thickened and slightly lemon-colored (about 3 minutes in a stand mixer, 5 minutes with a hand mixer.).

Slowly add oil, buttermilk, vanilla, and the coffee/melted chocolate mixture to the eggs, beating until just combined.
Add in the dry ingredient mixture on slow-to-medium speed until just combined.

Divide the batter evenly between the two prepared cake pans. Bake on the middle rack for 60-70 minutes, or until a toothpick or wooden skewer inserted in the center comes out clean.

Cool cake completely in pan on a wire rack. Run a thin knife around edges of pans and invert layers onto rack.

To make the ganache frosting, pour cream, sugar, and corn syrup into a medium-sized saucepan over medium heat, whisk constantly until simmering. Reduce heat to low and whisk in chocolate chips till melted. Remove from heat and whisk in the chopped butter. Try very, very hard to not eat this right now, all by itself. Cool frosting completely until it is glossy and of a spreadable consistency.

Spread frosting between cake layers and over the top and sides. If desired, top with mini chocolate chips. Serve chilled or at room temperature. Cake will keep covered and refrigerated for up to 3 days.

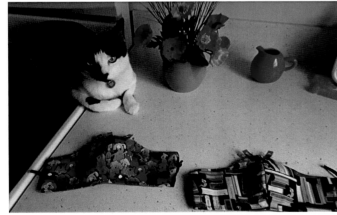

Photo Courtesy of Barbara Biro

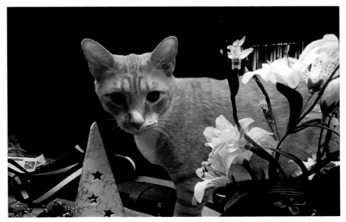

Photo Courtesy of Valerie Brown

Espresso Cherry Brownies

Chocolate and cherries, chocolate and coffee, chocolate and you – some things just belong together. I was thinking that as I opened a big box of dried Montmorency cherries shipped to me from Door County, WI by Grandma Jacque. If you've never been to Door County, please go. It's beautiful in any season, but it's nirvana for cherry lovers from mid-July to mid-August. You can pick your own which is so much fun, and lots of the orchards also sell jams, and wine, and some of the best cherry pies you will ever, ever taste. These brownies are for grownups: rich and dark, studded with sweet-tart dried cherries, bits of chocolate, and even a decent hit of caffeine from the espresso. My best friend hates chocolate – I know, I know – but loves these. I just about cried when she had seconds. I make these with cocoa powder instead of melted chocolate because 1) cocoa powder can survive the night in this house but chocolate isn't safe, and 2) texture. Cocoa powder makes for a more tender brownie which works well with the slightly chewy cherries.

1 cup all-purpose flour	2 cups dried cherries
2 cups white sugar	2 sticks butter, melted
4 large eggs	3 tsp espresso powder OR instant coffee powder*
¾ cup unsweetened cocoa powder	2 tsp pure vanilla extract
½ tsp baking powder	¾ cup dark or semi-sweet mini chocolate chips
¼ tsp salt	

Heat oven to 350°. Grease a 13x9x2 Nick & Joni's Cathead Biscuits baking pan (optional: line the bottom of the pan with parchment paper for easier removal and cleanup).

In a small bowl, whisk together flour, baking powder, and salt; set aside.

Using a large bowl, add espresso powder and vanilla extract to the melted butter. Stir in sugar. Add the eggs, one at a time, gently beating with a large spoon to combine. (You can do all of this by hand – no mixer required.) Stir in the cocoa powder until fully blended. Fold in the remaining dry ingredients. Add the dried cherries and mini chocolate chips.

Bake for 30 minutes. (An overbaked brownie is a dry, tragic thing so start checking for doneness a few minutes before the timer goes off. Look for the edges of the brownie to start pulling away from the sides of the pan, and for a toothpick inserted in the center to have a few moist crumbs but NO liquid batter.) Allow to cool in pan for at least an hour before slicing and serving. Yields 24.

*if you adore the flavor of coffee and caffeine doesn't make you twitch, you can increase espresso powder to 4 tsp.

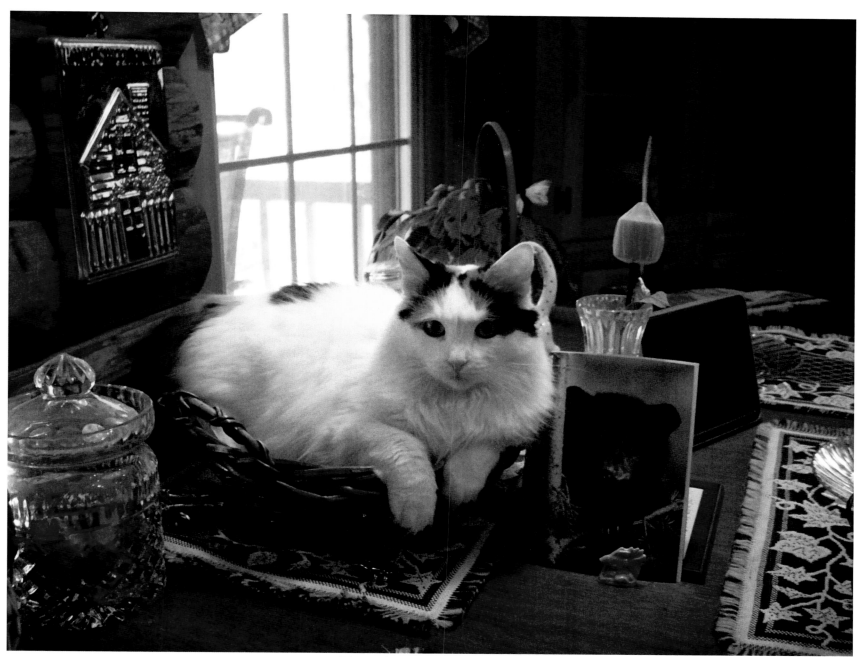

Photo Courtesy of Bill Zeeh

Alena's Chocolate Chip Cookies

Some cat ladies are born, some are made, and some just happen to have painstakingly perfected the most delicious chocolate chip cookies ever to come out of your oven. Alena's interest in cooking began at age 5 when she'd happily sit for hours and watch the Food Network. Now she's grown up, a newlywed, and a baking professional at a doughnut shop in California. "Learning new methods every day at work has inspired me to want to create recipes that are all my own, recipes I can someday give my children and grandchildren. Chocolate chip cookies are one of my favorites! I've made them every chance I could for years, and after many trials, I enjoy these more than any I've baked in the past." Added bonus: what's cuter than wee paw prints in the flour on your kitchen counters? "ANYTHING is cuter than that!" scream the non-cat people. Oh, hush now and have a cookie. Alena really knows her stuff and a few paw prints are the least of your worries. Truly.

1 ½ cups all-purpose flour
½ cup salted butter, softened
⅔ cup brown sugar, packed
⅓ cup granulated sugar
2 tsp vanilla extract
½ tsp baking powder

¼ tsp salt
1 large egg, room temperature
¼ tsp cinnamon
½ tsp lemon juice
½ cup semi-sweet chocolate chunks
½ cup milk chocolate chips

Whisk together flour, baking powder, salt, and cinnamon.

Using a stand or hand mixer, cream together butter and both sugars until light and fluffy – about 3 minutes.

Add egg, lemon juice, and vanilla, and beat until fluffy. Add in flour mixture, a third at a time, mixing until just incorporated. Using a spatula, gently fold in chocolate chunks and chocolate chips. Chill dough for 30 minutes.

Preheat oven to 350°. Line a cookie sheet with parchment paper.

Using a ¼ cup measure, shape dough into balls, and barely press down on center. Place cookies 4 inches apart, and bake for 12 minutes, until edges are golden brown. Let cookies sit on pan for 5 minutes and then enjoy while still hot OR move to a wire rack to cool completely. Yields 12 cookies.

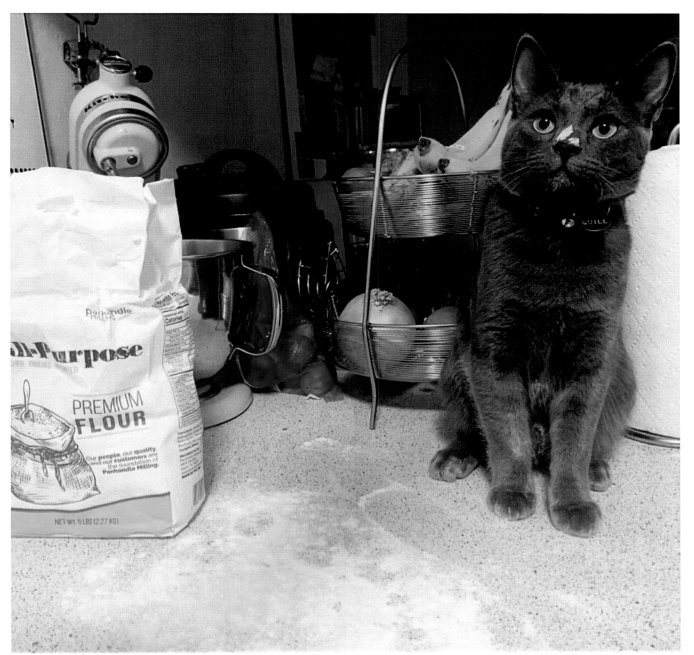

Photo Courtesy of Alena Schneider

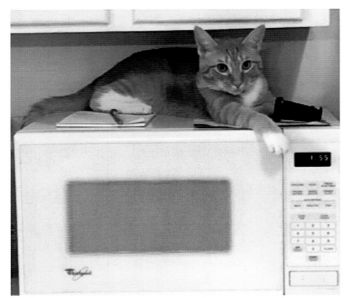

Photo Courtesy of Chris Wilson

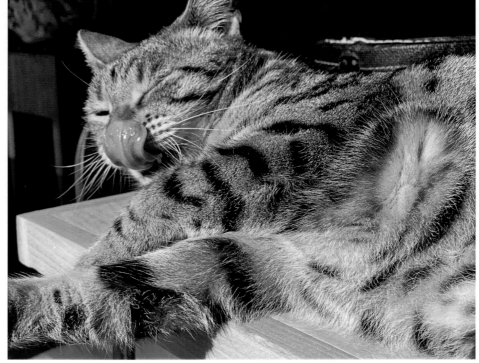

Photo Courtesy of Sheri Lynch

A Little Treat for Kitty

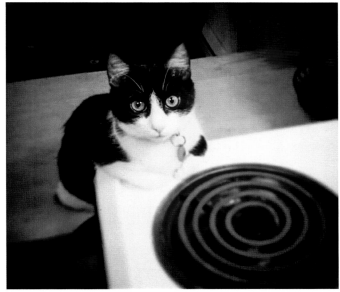

Photo Courtesy of Amanda Pierce

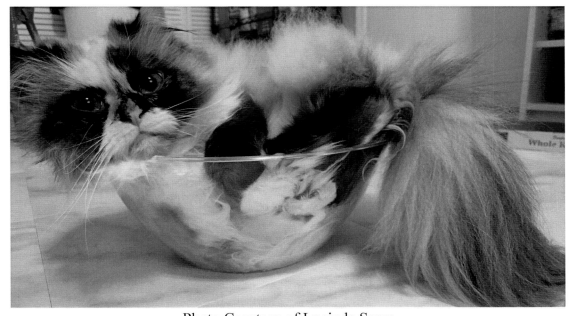

Photo Courtesy of Lucinda Sears

Kit Kat Snack Attack & Amews Bouche

You didn't think a book called *Cooking With Cats* would forget to whip up something yummy for the cats? Not a chance. These decadent little nibbles were created by a true cat empress, a woman astride her own multigenerational cat dynasty. Gina Whitt was volunteering at her local city animal shelter, working in the kitten nursery when a tiny baby with a fluff of curly gray fur was brought in. At just a couple of weeks old, he needed special care. Gina brought him home as a foster. Her grandson, Tucker, immediately declared that he wanted this kitten for his upcoming 13th birthday. So, Gina taught Tucker and his mom how to bottle feed and toilet train their new baby. It turned out that, tiny as he was, this kitten was capable of putting out quite a stench. Tucker jokingly began calling him "Stinky Pete" – classic 13 year-old boy stuff. The name mostly stuck and today Tinky Pete has an adoring family. Sadly, he lost his curls. But his grandma Gina makes treats for him that rival the appetizers served to guests at some weddings I've been to. Okay, well, some of my weddings anyway. Tinky Pete is a lucky cat, and a reminder that rescue might just be the greatest way to find your own kitty best friend.

Kit Kat Snack Attack

1 cup finely ground Instinct Raw Kibble   1 tbsp catnip
  (include the freeze-dried yummy bits)   Oil (Gina uses grapeseed oil)
1 5.5 oz can Fromm Salmon & Tuna Pate

Preheat the oven to 325°.

Combine first 3 ingredients to form a thick batter. Lightly grease your hands with oil, or your rolling pin, and pat or roll out the batter to 1/8-1/4 inch thickness. Cut into fun shapes of your choice and place on lightly oiled cookie sheet. Bake 10-12 minutes, or until crunchy. Baking this catnip concoction will bring all of the felines racing to the kitchen!

Amews Bouche

1 tube Inaba Churu Chicken Puree   15-20 tips of OurPets Kitty Cat Grass
5 large flakes of Cat Sushi Bonito flakes   5 spoons

Squeeze a lovely dollop of Inaba Churu onto each of the 5 spoons. Poke a large flake of Cat Sushi into the very top of each dollop so it stands upright. Stick 3 OurPets Grass tips – whiskers – into the side of each dollop. Serve only to the most discriminating of cats. With your pinkie held out, of course.

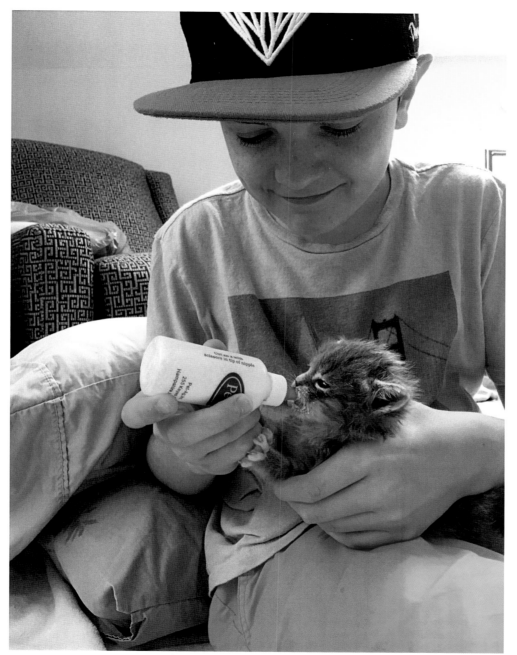

Photo Courtesy of Gina Whitt

Acknowledgments

Cooking with Cats was born when I jokingly told a friend that my next book was going to be a cookbook for crazy cat people. That friend, Tony Garcia, pretended it wasn't a joke and gave me a deadline. And here we are. (Check out Tony's recipe for Arroz Con Pollo a la Anubis). Thanks to Tony for his encouragement and help in getting this whole thing made. Thanks also to Heather Furr for the heroic job of pulling together so many amazing photos of cats wilding in kitchens. Every photo in this book was shared with us by a cat-loving *Bob & Sheri* listener. Hosting the *Bob & Sheri* radio show is my day job, and the people who listen are pretty much the best people you'll find anywhere. Plus, they love cats and they love food, which is a glorious combination. I'm grateful to everyone who offered a recipe: Jennifer Blackwell, Jane McNeely-Sowell, Mary Lacey, Joni Nash Case, Anne Oberlander, Courtney Armstrong, Kerri Green, Cynthia Conrow, Rick Sullivan, Jacque Axland, Alena Schneider, Jenn Jackson, Gina Whitt. I also want to shout out the wonderful cooks in our family who are shooing cats off the counters in that big kitchen in the sky: Sarah Nash, Jewel Sullivan, Isabel Bartholetti, Rena Lynch, Rosemary Whalen. I must also thank my mom for being my first cat lady role model, that Easy Bake Oven, and the recipe for her mother's meatballs (Italians do not part with such things lightly). There are so many home cooks I've watched and learned from, including my beloved sister-in-law, Nancy Lynch, and my college boyfriend's grandmother, Mrs. Speranza, who once made a meal to rival anything I've eaten in Italy in a makeshift kitchen tucked into a spare bedroom in her son's home in Philly.

I worked on *Cooking with Cats* during the Covid-19 pandemic, so my family may remember this challenging period as the Taste This Era. Leah Nash – along with Andrew and baby Ada - really stepped up and cheerfully sampled version after version of Espresso Cherry Brownies and Pumpkin Spice Lovers Bread. My awesome besties, Evelyn Warren and Rick Sullivan, were held hostage while I figured out savory tarts, apple cakes, and a handful of others that didn't make the cut. My sister-wife Joni Nash Case (she used to be married to my husband, but now she's mine because that man clearly has a type) offered much love and encouragement and, along with Jane McNeely-Sowell, all sorts of fun cat-centric ideas. Speaking of my husband, Kevin is not at all a foodie and doesn't like sweets (which is super disturbing), but he happily ate every version of every recipe and is always on board and supportive of whatever insane plan I come up with next. I've been food-experimenting on my daughters, Olivia and Caramia, since the day they were born and they're both great sports about it. Olivia is already a terrific, creative cook and Caramia is a skilled baker. They learned by hanging out and helping in the kitchen and I know that the long line of women who came before them are watching from beyond with delight and pride. Big thanks to Bob Lacey, Todd Haller, and Max Sweeten. They didn't cook anything or clean up anything, but I love them like brothers and they always have my back: on-air, off-air, in the kitchen, and everywhere. Finally, thank YOU for reading. I hope you found something in here that you'll want to make again and again. A portion of the proceeds of this book are being donated to help cats not lucky enough to be roaming your kitchen, stealing bites, cared for and loved.

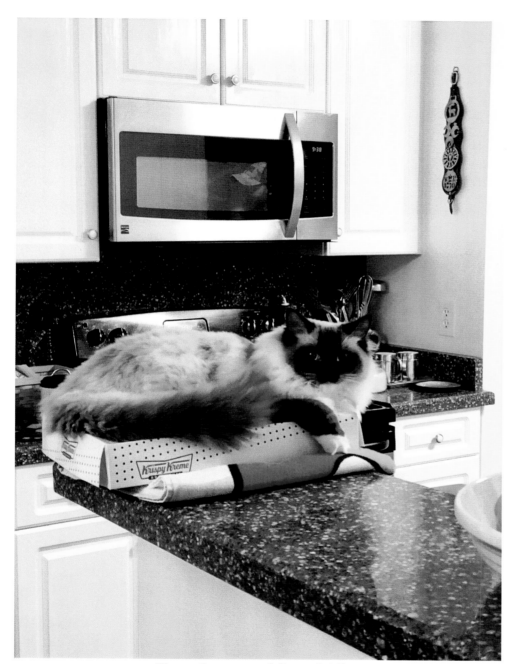

Photo Courtesy of Crystal Allen

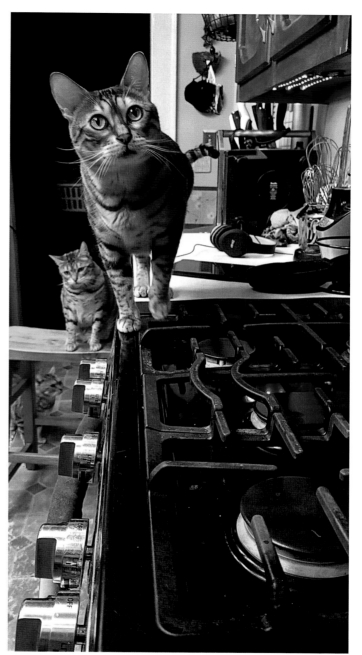

Photo Courtesy of Kimberly Robinson

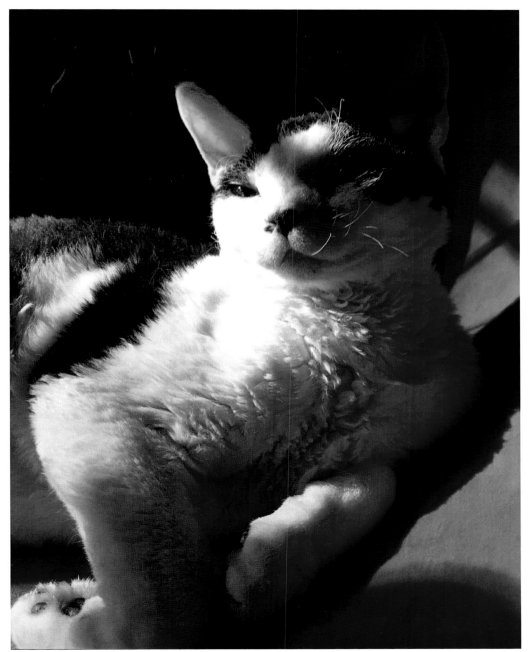

Photo Courtesy of Sheri Lynch